Behind the Old Face

Aging in America and the Coming Elder Boom

Priscilla,
God Bless
You + Your
Family,
Love
Angil

By Angil Tarach-Ritchey RN, GCM

DreamSculpt Media Inc.
Sonoma, CA. USA

ISBN 978-1-937504-33-5
DSP 104

For more information, visit
www.DreamSculpt.com
info@DreamSculpt.com

Book and cover design by Darlene Swanson of Van-garde Imagery, Inc.

Produced and distributed for DreamSculpt Media, Inc.
by BackOffice Publisher Services, Worthy Shorts, Inc.

Dedication

I dedicate this book to the Lord, for giving me the passion, ability, knowledge, gifts, talents, experiences, and work I love. I am grateful and humbled to be used for this work and know that without God this would not be possible. My life has been truly blessed by the time I have spent with seniors and being able to provide care and assistance. To God I give all the glory!

I also dedicate this book to every senior who has ever been treated disrespectfully, without dignity, been neglected or abused. With you in mind, I have committed my life to advocacy, and doing what I can to prevent mistreatment of as many aging adults as possible.

In memory of my grandma,
Veronica Kwiatkowski,
who is deeply missed and holds
a very special place in my heart.

Contents

Part 3   The Future of Aging

Part 1   The Current Climate of Aging

Chapter 1
The Nursing Home Love Letters
My story in the nursing home

What would you title a defining moment in your life, the moment that changed everything? My earliest defining moment came in a box of love letters. No, not letters to me. It all happened with a box of love letters I found in a nursing home.

My love for the elderly began when I started working as an aide in a nursing home in 1977, when I was seventeen years old. My girlfriend's mother, Mrs. Berry, was a registered nurse and the nursing home administrator. She was a tall, fairly thin woman with blonde hair. Although Mrs. Berry was "cool" most of the time, it was apparent when she was angry or had enough with teenagers in her home. She would make it clear she'd had enough just by the look on her face. I liked Mrs. Berry and respected her, but I also feared her. I never knew if she really liked me or not. Her daughter, my friend Marcy, worked for her mom at the nursing home as a nurse's aide. She would tell us stories about the residents at her job, and most of the stories were amusing. I needed a job, so I thought I could do what Marcy was doing. I approached Mrs. Berry several times asking for a job. I think she was passively ignoring me, but I was persistent . . . when Mrs. Berry was in a good mood, that is. After a month or two of asking her repeatedly to hire me and give me a chance, she finally agreed with the comment, "I'll give you a chance, but I don't think you can do it." What

Mrs. Berry didn't know was that I am highly motivated by disbelief. I have accomplished more in my lifetime because people told me I couldn't do something than because people told me I could.

It was a warm, humid day in June 1977, and I was about to begin my first job as a nurse's aide. When I arrived at the nursing home at 7:00 a.m., never having cared for an elderly person before, I assumed there would be some sort of formal training. My training was to follow another aide around, and basically do what she did. I wanted to follow Marcy, because we were friends and her mom ran the place, but Mrs. Berry wouldn't allow that. I know she expected we would be goofing off or doing some kind of foolishness if we worked together, so she had me follow a nurse's aide I had never met. I have to say, I was a little intimidated by the ninety or so residents, some walking through the halls with canes and walkers, some being wheeled down the hall in wheelchairs, and others yelling or talking to themselves. But I had to prove to Mrs. Berry I could do it, so I just took it minute by minute. There was no way I would confirm her notion that I couldn't do the work.

My first day seemed to be a test of my physical and emotional endurance. I worked sixteen hours that day, and within a few hours on the job I was involved in a medical emergency. We were passing lunch trays when the whole room turned chaotic in response to a resident choking on her lunch. The whole situation seemed to be happening in slow motion, even though it only lasted a few short minutes. I realized the resident was choking, because her table mates were yelling and I saw her gripping her throat. Since it was my first day and I was not ready for a situation like this, I looked around the room to make sure an employee knew what was going on and would react. I had never expected to see something like this, especially on my first day of work. As my eyes quickly scanned the room,

I saw my supervisor frozen in position, fear evident on her face. The experienced nurse's aides were either screaming for someone to do something or trying to ignore the urgency of the situation.

Residents began yelling and getting out of their seats, waiting and watching for someone to help her. It seemed everyone was waiting for someone else to react, and no one was moving towards her. As seconds passed, her face started turning blue. I just knew if no one helped her, she would die. I had never received training for the Heimlich maneuver, or any other formal training, but when she began turning blue and no one acted or seemed to know what to do, I knew I had to do something. I could not watch this woman die in front of me without doing something! I remembered seeing the Heimlich maneuver done on TV and figured I had to try it. I ran to the table and grabbed her now lifeless, thin body and pulled her against my chest. I clenched my fists around her tiny waist and forcefully pulled her upper abdomen toward me. I pulled once, twice, and finally the third time she coughed out the food that was lodged in her throat. Her body then regained life, and her blue skin began changing back to a light pink pigment. She was going to be okay. I was flooded with emotions: disbelief, shock, fear, relief, gratitude, anger, and pride. Of course, I was relieved and grateful, but I was angry that my supervisor had no idea what to do and didn't even attempt to help this lady. I wondered how she could be the person in charge. I wondered what would have happened to this lady if I hadn't at least tried the Heimlich maneuver or if it hadn't worked. The truth is, I was not sure I could do anything to help. I was in shock and petrified that I was going to see someone die right in front of my eyes. This was a lot more than I had bargained for when I asked Mrs. Berry to give me a chance. After the adrenalin dissipated, I felt very proud for having saved the resident's life and that I had lost the intimidation I felt just minutes earlier. I also lost respect for a supervisor I barely knew. This was my initiation into senior care and advocacy.

The facility was supposed to support independent to semi-independent living, which today we refer to as assisted living. There were three floors: the first floor residents were independent; the second floor residents were mostly semi-independent with a few dependent residents; and the third floor housed all the residents who shouldn't have been living there. I believe it was set up that way so when visitors or potential new residents' families came, they would see the very best in independent living. There were no tours beyond the first floor to my recollection. I continued working as a nurse's aide on the afternoon shift. I was responsible for all of the residents on the third floor.

My residents were either totally physically dependent, or had Alzheimer's or some other form of dementia. Back then we described a person with dementia as being senile. My responsibilities were to keep my incontinent residents clean, to get everyone to the dining room for their dinner and medications, to pass dinner trays, and to feed those who could not feed themselves. I was also responsible for entertaining the residents after dinner, which meant sitting them in the day room to watch TV while I cleaned up dinner trays and tables, changed residents, gave baths, and started getting residents ready for bed.

The day shift was responsible for half of the residents' baths and grooming each week, and I was responsible for the other half. I was the only aide on the third floor afternoon shift. I don't recall how many residents I had to care for; I just remember it was a lot of work. I had responsibilities and experiences on this job I never would have imagined: shaving a man with a non-electric razor; being with a person with dementia; cleaning an incontinent person; tying people to their beds to keep them safe from falling; feeding an adult; and, convincing someone to take a bath when they refused.

There was no training to teach me how to do these tasks or to deal with dementia patients. Nurse's aides were just hired and put to work, until 1987 when Congress passed the Omnibus Reconciliation Act, commonly referred to as OBRA. Safety concerns and the lack of quality care in our nation's nursing homes inspired OBRA, which required training nursing home staff. Talk about old school; I was doing this work for ten years before the U.S. required training.

One night, a few months into my job, I started my shift looking through the bath book to see who was scheduled for a bath. I also looked through the documentation from the day shift. There were residents on the day-shift schedule who hadn't had a bath in a month or more. I was outraged and saddened. I gave thirty-two baths in one night. I worked a couple of hours of overtime to get it all done, but all the residents on the third floor were now clean and cared for. Was this the first night of a lifetime of senior advocacy? Looking back over thirty years, I think it was. I couldn't understand how anyone could let this happen. The residents were people, and they needed help. What if these lazy nurse's aides were deprived a bath for a month? What would they want?

I had no idea at the time how significant the bath night and another experience I had would become in how I have spent my life caring and advocating for seniors. The experiences clearly had their own purposes. One began my life as a senior advocate; the other was the major contributing factor to the empathetic care I have provided all of my life. Thirty years later, there are many patients I still remember, think about, and hold dear to my heart. I remember a retired teacher who had dementia and filed things in her bra. She said they were her files, as if she were still teaching. I remember a couple who walked the halls holding hands; the husband wore the layers of men's and women's clothing his wife dressed him in. I remember a tall thin lady with dementia, who was either glowingly joyful while singing in her high-pitched, out-of-tune voice or so angry she hit and scratched anyone who came near her. I can still picture these residents clearly, and I hold fond memories of them in my heart.

One evening, our assignment was to clean our residents' closets and drawers. One of my residents was a lady named Ann, who couldn't speak or do anything for herself. She quietly lay in bed day after day. Ann never had a visitor, so I knew nothing about her. While I was working in Ann's room, I found a box in her closet. In it were no less than thirty letters and cards. I sat on the floor and started to read them, one after another, as tears fell from my eyes. They were love letters from a husband to his wife. Never had I known, or even heard about, such profound and amazing love. This woman, lying there alone seemingly unloved, had actually shared a fairy-tale love, rare and amazing, with an adoring spouse. I can still vividly recall sitting on the floor with her box in my lap, tears dripping from my face, reading the letters while frequently pausing to look at Ann lying in that bed, almost lifeless, wishing I had known her sooner.

I wished I knew about her life when I started caring for her. For many months, I had looked at her as just some old woman lying in the bed who needed help. Truthfully, until that day I didn't give her much thought other than the duties of keeping her clean, dry, and physically comfortable. Not that I didn't occasionally think how sad it was she never had a visitor or any indication that someone cared about her, but that was the extent of my thoughts and involvement with her. Before I left my shift that night, I acknowledged Ann. She was no longer just some old woman. I went to her, and while gently stroking her cheek and forehead I said, "Your husband sure did love you." I said goodnight and went home. That was all I could say, given the emotional state I was in after reading all those letters. I'm not sure if I was more sad about Ann's loss and being alone in that nursing home or guilty for not seeing her as a real person with a real life.

It was through her letters that I got to know Ann, who couldn't tell me any-thing about herself. As far as I knew, her deceased husband was all she had, and now I felt more responsibility to take care of her for him. That was when the meaning of care changed for me. Previous to this night, I felt that I pro-vided pretty good care given the number of residents I had and the duties that needed to be done. I kept Ann clean and dry, but I didn't know how to communicate with someone who couldn't acknowledge me or speak back. Although I gave good physical care, there was no emotion involved, no hu-man connection; I was very quiet when I provided care for Ann.

I now had something to talk to Ann about. Caring for Ann changed into something much more meaningful. I felt a special bond with her. Those love letters gave me much deeper empathy for my residents. I started look-ing at all of the residents, wondering what lives they previously had before they ended up in that nursing home. That revelation inspired me to find out as much as I could about them. I read their charts, asked questions, listened to their conversations more intently, and observed their actions. From time to time, I would read Ann's husband's letters to her. I don't know whether Ann could understand or even hear anything I said, but I felt that her spirit heard and understood. I also felt as if her husband was looking down from heaven, grateful for someone who was telling Ann about his love in a comforting and caring way and taking care of her physically.

Ann's inability to speak was due to aphasia, a speech and language disorder that impairs a person's ability to communicate It is most commonly the re-sult of a stroke but can occur from any severe head injury and affects over one million people in the U.S. Aphasia can be expressive, meaning the per-son can fully comprehend language but cannot verbally express thoughts, feelings, or preferences. Aphasia can also be receptive, meaning patients can't understand verbal or written language. People often assume that a per-son with expressive aphasia cannot understand or comprehend, but that is far from the truth. Not knowing whether Ann had receptive aphasia, I truly don't know if she understood me when I talked to her and read her love letters to her. But, I think there is something in our souls that allows us to connect even when the typical means of communication are not possible.

My three-decade passion has been based on empathy. Can you imagine being in Ann's shoes? Can you understand what it must be like to have lived a fairy-tale life with a best friend, experience a love like no other, only to lose that person and decline to the point where you are alone and unable to care for yourself? I don't know if it was true or not, but I heard Ann's decline was a result of losing her husband. We often hear about couples who have been married for many years dying close in time, so her decline following the loss of her husband wouldn't surprise me.

Ann's is just one story in a countless numbers of stories. There are thousands of elders living in nursing homes, alone and unable to care for themselves. What kind of care do they get when their healthcare workers know nothing about them and don't even think about what their lives were like before they ended up helpless and in a nursing home? Just like I did. I've worked in long-term care for decades and never saw any training programs that focused on communicating with persons with aphasia, or even explained what it is. I also have never seen any training programs that elicited empathy—other than The Virtual Dementia Tour®, which provides a great learning experience. I know from my own experience that patients like Ann are not spoken to or treated with the compassion that is essential to providing good care. Instead, they're regarded as work to be done rather than a person to whom care is given. It is up to us as a society to understand that there is a person and a life Behind the Old Face.

In over three decades of spending time caring and advocating for seniors, many experiences brought me to write this book, but a single experience at a funeral home inspired the idea and title; I share that experience with you later in this chapter. Throughout this book, I will share my experiences and the stories of a few of the seniors I have spent time with, but my experiences and their stories provide only a small glimpse of what is Behind the Old Face. This book is intended to tug at your heart strings, to make anyone interacting with or caring for an elderly person think differently, and to subsequently improve the way we treat seniors and the care we provide. Care should never be just a physical-care task. Anyone can provide physical care, but great care providers offer an emotional component to their care that makes it great. There are unpaid caregivers, such as family, friends, and volunteers, as well as a wide range of paid caregivers, including nurse's aides, therapists, nurses, social workers, and physicians. No paid care giving job is more important than another. No care recipient is more important than another. Whatever your care giving role, you need to provide care with respect, compassion, empathy, and kindness. All care recipients should always—without exception—be treated with dignity, respect, and from an empathetic point of view.

Every single one of us has heard, "Treat people as you want to be treated," but how many of us really do? How many nurse's aides, nurses, physicians, and family caregivers provide the treatment they would want to receive? Do you treat every single person you come in contact with, have a relationship with, work with, or care for as you would want to be treated?

As you read this book and the stories of the people in it, you will and should experience a myriad of emotions. I will tell you some of the most amazing stories I have ever heard, from the lives of seniors I have been privileged to know and spend time with. These aren't famous people with amazing newsworthy stories; these are everyday stories. These are the life stories of your parents, grandparents, neighbors, aunts and uncles, the old man driving too slow, the grey-haired old woman that you have to wait on in the store, the patient you have to feed or change, the Alzheimer's patient who is difficult, and the dementia patient who asks the same questions over and over. These people are us. They are us, with many more years of life behind them. You will hear about their challenges, their dreams achieved or not achieved, their contributions and accomplishments, their service to our country or to a cause, their devastations and joys, their thoughts, feelings, and opinions, and their points of view about what it's like to be a senior today.

Even after my decades of spending time with seniors, I still hear things that are surprising to me, and things I have never thought of. While interviewing one lady for the book, she told me a secret. At her request, I will not use her name or feature her story in the book, but she told me something that gave me another perspective into things that seniors think about. She was a lovely ninety-one-year old woman I'll call Susan. Susan grew up in England, and even years after being in America, she still had a lovely English accent. I cared for her while her husband was in the hospital. She was happily married for over seventy years, and she adored her husband. During interviews, I ask specific questions to initiate further conversation and to better understand what it's like to be old. One question I ask is, "Who is your hero?" When I asked Susan this question, she said it was her husband, but as we continued to talk about her life from childhood on, she asked, "Can I tell you a secret?"

Susan started talking about her first love when she was nineteen. Her blue eyes sparkled as she told me about their weekends spent dancing at a local hangout. He was a very handsome man, a man of honor and values, who could dance "as gracefully as Fred Astaire," she said in a giddy, schoolgirl-crush way. They were together a few months when he went into the military. While he was away, she met her husband. You may think the rest is history, but it wasn't. Her entire life, she had thought about her first love and how things may have been different if she had waited for him. Imagine spending seventy-two years thinking about a lost love and the what-if's.

Susan described times they would run into each other after he returned from the military and she was already another man's wife. They had an un-spoken bond they both recognized and possibly even longed for. She de-scribed the small bits of conversation they had and said he would always ask, "Are you okay, Susan? Really? He never married, and Susan won-dered if it was because he wanted to marry her. She thought his "Really?" carried an undertone of a deeper question. Susan thought he wanted to know if she was truly happy with another man as her husband. He was too much of a gentleman to get between Susan and her husband, so she felt there were words that were never spoken. They eventually lost track of each other because of her move to the U.S.

Her secret revealed that she never let the memories or the what-if's go. She kept them quietly stored away in her heart for over seventy years. It was a heartwarming story. I felt a bit sad hearing it. I was sitting with a wonderful woman of ninety-one who had never gotten over her first love. I was honored that I was the first one she had ever told this to. I was also surprised by what I had been told. Susan went on to tell me how wonder-ful her husband had always been to her and how she never regretted mar-rying him. She kept her thoughts secret her whole life so as not to hurt her husband, who was her hero.

We talked about her life over the course of a couple days. She shared her experiences as an elderly woman in the hospital. Susan described an ex-perience during one of her hospital admissions. A couple of nurses mim-icked her accent. This had happened years before we met, yet had stayed in her thoughts and feelings. Susan described feeling disrespected, belittled, and treated as if she had no feelings. The mimicking nurses made her feel like they thought she was stupid because she had an accent. I would guess there was no mal intent on the part of the nurses, but they didn't think about Susan's dignity or feelings either.

As you progress through this book and read about the lives of the people described in it, you will read about situations that will warm your heart and others that are disturbing. Both are intended to cause you to think, put yourself in someone else's shoes, and move you to a more compassionate perspective when it comes to our elders. It is my hope that the stories will be heartwarming enough to cause you to be kinder and more thoughtful, and disturbing enough to inspire you to become an advocate for better treatment of one of our most vulnerable populations.

Funerals reveal who we have been

In my work and life, I have been to countless funerals, home viewings, and memorial ceremonies. Funerals can be as unique as the individual who died, but in the last ten to fifteen years, I have noticed increasing numbers of families inviting loved ones and friends to share memories. Shared memories give attendees more knowledge about the deceased person and offer perspectives that are sometimes unknown even to spouses or best friends. Personally, this is my favorite part of a funeral.

No funeral has stood out more to me than the one I attended for Brad Houghtalin. Brad was a man in his fifties and the son of the late Carlton Houghtalin. Brad and his dad lived together until a few days before Brad died. In December 2002, I received a call from Ron Houghtalin inquiring about homecare services for his dad, Carlton. Ron lives in Washington and his dad lived in Michigan. Ron told me his brother, Brad, lived with his Dad and had been caring for him but had some health issues of his own, and caring for their dad was becoming too much for Brad. I set up an appointment to meet Carlton and Brad, and to assess Carlton's needs.

When I arrived at their home, I found Brad to be a very pleasant but rather shy man and Carlton to be grumbling a bit about my visit and the proposal of outside help. I like working with gruff, outspoken clients. I'm not sure if it's because I am an outspoken type myself or because I learned years back in that nursing home at seventeen that I could get the residents who refused baths or meals to do as I wanted them to. Needless to say, Carlton was going to be a great challenge. Ron had informed me that Brad had a seizure disorder so that our care team would be aware and not call an ambulance the first time we observed a seizure.

We agreed to begin some part-time services assisting Carlton with hygiene, grooming, and meal preparation. My homecare agency prided itself on introducing the caregivers in advance so clients become comfortable with them. Brad and Carlton didn't feel the need for a meeting to introduce caregivers prior to our start date, so I planned to meet the first caregiver at their home on the first day to introduce her and acclimate her to the home and the plan of care before leaving her to work her shift.

I wasn't five minutes away when the caregiver called me, a bit frantic, because Brad was having a seizure. We provide nonmedical care, so this was not something our caregivers were trained or experienced in handling. As a nurse with much experience caring for patients with epilepsy, I calmed her and stayed with her on the phone as I guided her through the steps to make sure Brad was safe from injury. This was the first of many seizures Brad had when we were in the home providing service to his dad.

When we started working with the Houghtalins in 2002, my agency had been open only four months. I had a lot of available time in those days to spend visiting our clients. Because neither Brad nor Carlton drove, I felt they were socially deprived and I visited often. I got to know them and the whole family well as time went on. The only friends Brad ever talked about were a lesbian couple who often visited him. I never met them, but Brad talked about how much he enjoyed their friendship and visits.

As far as I knew, they were the only friends Brad had. He and Carlton had visits only from family, the lady friends, and people from my agency. I would stop by with snacks and chat or bring Brad some movies, and they seemed to enjoy my visits. I was always happy to see them and felt like I was bringing some of the outside in. Brad and Carlton had not been eating particularly well on their own, so we included meal preparation in our services. I believe they enjoyed the food and also the company of the cooks.

Ron and his now-late wife, Nancy, came into town as often as possible, and we would meet for breakfast or lunch. Susan, Ron's cousin and a registered nurse, took care of Carlton's doctor appointments, medications, and anything else of a medical nature. She lived nearby and visited frequently. The whole family was wonderful, and we all became good friends. The Houghtalin family exuded love and were always concerned for each other, helping in any way they could if someone in their family was in need.

In 2005, as months passed, Carlton had more health problems. He was in and out of the hospital and seemed to decline a little bit more with every hospitalization. One morning, it seemed I visited at the perfect time, because Brad and my agency caregiver were trying to wake Carlton up and he wasn't responding. He was a non-insulin diabetic, and his blood sugar had dropped so low during the night that he was in a hypoglycemic crisis. Brad and my caregiver were not experienced enough to recognize the cause of Carlton's nonresponsive symptoms, so I was very grateful I arrived when I did. I put some grape jam under Carlton's tongue, and he soon started waking up. When he was alert enough to swallow, we gave him some juice and fed him a good breakfast. I don't think I ever told Ron about that incident, because it would have worried him more, and as far away as he was, he would have felt more helpless. I gave clear instructions to Brad and to my staff about Carlton's nutritional needs and the signs and symptoms of low and high blood sugar.

The family was aware of most everything else, and as Carlton continued to decline, Ron asked us to increase care from part-time to full-time and eventually to live-in. In November of that year, the family decided that it was all too much for Brad, and that Carlton needed to be watched more closely, so they decided to move him to Susan's home at the beginning of the year. In December, Carlton was again hospitalized. The family decided he would go to Susan's following his discharge, since it was so close to the beginning of the year anyway. Ron wanted to retain our services on a regular basis at Susan's home to give her respite time and so she could continue her church involvement and spend time with her grandchildren.

The caregivers and I were a bit sad we wouldn't see Brad on a regular basis but understood their decision to move Carlton. Brad's seizures seemed to be increasing as well, but stress often brings on more frequent seizures. We all assumed the seizures would lessen without the stress of worrying about his dad and dealing with caregivers coming and going.

We weren't out of the home a week when I got one of the most shocking phone calls I'd ever received. On New Year's Day 2006, Ron called me to tell me that Brad had died. Huh? Brad? Did he mean Carlton? No, he did say Brad. I held the phone in disbelief. A call saying Carlton had passed away would have been just as sad, but it would have been much more expected. Ron told me that from what he gathered, Brad was in the basement when he had a seizure and died. As a previous hospice nurse who has dealt so much with death, I don't usually cry at the news of a death.

It's not that I am not sad or feel bad for the family, it's just that most of the people I've cared for who have died were much older and were expected to die. Brad wasn't one of those people. I took his death harder than I thought I would. I wondered then and still wonder now, if we were still providing live-in services in his home, would we have been able to call emergency services and save Brad? I'll never know the answer.

The day of Brad's funeral arrived. My sister and I went together. She was my agency's assistant director at the time and also got to know and love this family. I expected it to be a small, quiet funeral with family, a few friends, and us. When we approached the funeral home, we could hardly get into the parking lot because there were so many people. Since funeral homes sometimes have more than one service going on, we assumed the traffic was for someone else's service. We walked in and asked the funeral home director where to find Brad. We were directed towards a room that was overflowing with people; there were so many people, they were standing shoulder-to-shoulder and flowing out into the hallway.

We made our way through the room, looking at one unfamiliar face after another, until we spotted Carlton sitting in his wheelchair in the front row with our caregiver at his side. We hugged him, extending our condolences. His face appeared older and his eyes were more distant than before. He whispered, "Thank you," and sat quietly, like he was in another world. I guess that losing a child no matter what age they are is like entering an unfamiliar world that no one ever wants to go to, and most of us never do. We stood silently there with Carlton, holding his hand and still looking around the room in disbelief. Who were all these people, friends of the family?

I spotted Ron standing a few feet away, chatting with mourners who came to express their sympathy. Ron met eyes with me, and I told Carlton I would be back. I thanked our caregiver for her attention to Carlton and went to hug Ron and express our sympathy. What do you say to the loved ones? I tend to say I am sorry for their loss or tell them I don't know what to say. Ron's wife Nancy made her way over to us, and we extended hugs and sympathy to her as well. Nancy had been struggling with health problems, just as I had been only to a more debilitating degree. I was surprised to see her using a walker since I hadn't seen her in awhile. I was thinking about how much this family had been through when Ron grabbed my hand to introduce me to his adopted brother.

Another shock for me! I never heard about an adopted brother. Apparently, he had heard of me, because he said so. I met a couple of other people introduced as foster children, now adults, of Carlton and his late wife Mary. Mary had died a few years prior, so unfortunately I never met her. I didn't know about any foster children either. Within forty minutes of entering the funeral home, I learned that Brad had been an incredible golf pro and had many friends and golf students who loved and respected him. I also learned that Carlton and Mary took in foster children and adopted one or two. I learned that Susan was Carlton's deceased brother's daughter and one of five nieces that Carlton and Mary took in to raise after his brother died. His nieces were young at the time; Carlton and Mary took all but the oldest.

As the funeral director started moving people to their seats so they could begin the service, I sat there in total shock about everything I had just learned. I thought I knew Brad and Carlton well, but I had no idea what kind of lives they led prior to my meeting them. I knew this family for just over three years at this point and assumed I knew all about them. Person after person got up and talked about memories of Brad and what he meant to them. We heard endearing stories, funny moments, and lots of expression of love and respect, but none tore at our emotions more than when Susan spoke of her dear Uncle Carlton who took the place of her dad when he died and of her life with Brad as her cousin and brother. As I listened to those who wanted to express their love and share memories, I thought about how humble great people are. In all the time I spent with Brad and Carlton, not once did Brad talk about golf, nor Carlton about his love for children and the sacrifices he and Mary made to raise them. I looked at Carlton sitting in the front row, looking so empty and sad, and in an instant the idea for this book and title, Behind the Old Face, entered my thoughts.

I thought about all the times Carlton was in and out of the hospital and the time a rehab center he was discharged to called me because he refused his meds. They heard I could get him to take his meds and asked me if I could help. I thought about the gentleness and goodness of a man who appeared so gruff on the outside and wondered how he was treated in the hospital and rehab facility. I wondered if he would have been treated differently had anyone known of the love and compassion he had for children. How humble he was; he never once mentioned it.

As I sat in that funeral home chair, I kept thinking about the gruff impression of Carlton's old face and how there was so much more behind his visual appearance. Hence, *Behind the Old Face.* Carlton's soft, loving, compassionate heart was not apparent on the outside. His sacrifice to children was not etched in his skin and because he was such a humble man, this wasn't something outsiders would know.

How often do any of us think we know someone or look into the face of an old person without ever thinking there is more? How often does anyone try to get to know the elderly patient in the hospital, the lady with dementia in the nursing home, or the combative man who refuses medications? Could you guess that a grumbling old man who doesn't want to be bothered or refuses to cooperate had such love in his heart and gave so much to improve the lives of children in need? Is the lack of joy in an old face due to loss of a spouse, loss of independence, or daily pain that cannot be relieved? Now that I think about Carlton in the fuller context of who he was, I believe Mary's passing and his loss of independence were more difficult for him than anyone knew. One thing I can happily say is that I loved that gruff old man before I knew the depths of him and his life.

I am thankful that I learned the lesson from Ann when I was young. I recognize there is more to a person even when I don't know what the "more" is. Even though Ann never said a word to me, she changed my life and the lives of every person I've cared for since. Without a doubt, Ann is the reason I spent a lifetime providing better care and became passionate about advocating for the improved treatment and care of the elderly. Whether or not a person is able to communicate or be an active participant in life, they can make a world of difference. I sometimes wonder if Ann is in heaven looking down on the impact she's made. I hope she knows just how special she was and how much better a person I became because of her.

What were your first memories of an elderly person?

Ann, Carlton, and Brad gave me notable lessons that changed what I think and how I provide care to aging adults. But they are not my earliest memories of elderly people. Apparently, I enjoyed spending time with elderly people since I was a very young girl. My first memory of an old person is probably that of my paternal grandfather. When I was born, up until I was three or four years old, we lived upstairs from my grandfather in an upper flat. He had a dog named Peppy. In the mornings, I went downstairs to see Grandpa and Peppy. Grandpa made coffee and bread. The coffee was sweet and filled with cream; we would dunk the bread in the coffee while we chatted. When we finished eating, Grandpa would take Peppy and me to the park. He'd push me on the swing or spin me on the merry-go-round. I was very young at the time, so I don't remember a lot of details, but I do remember Grandpa made me feel special, and his face would light up when I came into the room. He died when I was very young. I didn't understand it much at the time, and I barely recall that event. I have some 8mm movies of me tap dancing for Grandpa; it warms my heart when I watch them. My Dad still talks of how special I was to my Grandpa.

We moved around the time Grandpa died. An elderly couple lived next door to our new home. I loved to visit the lady next door and followed her around her house, chatting away as she tended to her garden or hung clothes to dry. Maybe she was a subconscious replacement for my grandpa, now that I think about it. A year or two after we moved in, my elderly friend went through a tragic and horrible experience, and so did I. Her husband poured gasoline all over her and their house, lit it, and the house blew up. He died the next day. She died three months later of pneumonia. I was very sad, because I felt like she was my friend.

Have you thought about your early experiences as you read about mine? Does a grandparent, family friend, neighbor, or someone else come to mind? You may feel warm and joyful feelings when you think about your first memories of an elderly person or you may feel anger, fear, dread, and even shame. I assumed our childhood experience with the elderly had more of a direct role in our individual attitudes and perceptions of the elderly than it directly does. Research in the *World Scientific Journal* in an article titled "Ageism: Does it Exist among Children?" states, "results indicate that a majority of children have positive perceptions and attitudes about old age, which leads us to the conclusion that ageism is adopted later in life." The findings encourage developing strategies to prevent formation of prejudices against elderly, which they agree is best achieved by intergenerational programs and education. Whether we expose children to time with aging adults because we believe it will contribute to a positive influence or prevent a negative one, it appears that intergenerational exposure has a positive influence over our later adult attitudes.

Some children don't have much, if any, experience with older adults until they enter their school years because they have no grandparents or their grandparents are distant. Our experiences are as different as we are. I truly can't say if the loving influence of my grandparents or my elderly neighbor had anything to do with my passion for eldercare and advocacy. I can only say for sure that I thought differently and my passion for eldercare and advocacy began when I had my experience with Ann.

The vast majority of us will not work as aides in nursing homes or spend a large amount of time with the elderly, but we all have thoughts and feelings when we come in contact with an old person. We have differing opinions of what we see and think is old. Our concept of old changes as we age ourselves. I remember as a young girl thinking that thirty or forty was old, and now I think one hundred is old! I know there are adults who look at an old person with disgust and others who look at them with respect. The problem is that there are too many who fall in the middle and don't think about old people much at all.

Can you think of times you were impatient or grumbled under your breath when you were held up by an old person? Maybe you have gone out of your way to help an elderly person who needed assistance. Would you? If you saw an elderly couple leaving a grocery store, one pushing the other in a wheelchair or helping them along with a walker, would you be the one to help them get their groceries in the car or walk by without considering lending a hand?

On a regular basis, you can find a senior shopping alone in a scooter or wheelchair, trying to get to a product off a shelf that is beyond their reach. Would you understand the difficulty of shopping from a wheelchair, or would you shy away because you don't recognize the need for assistance or you don't want to be bothered? An episode of a TV program called *What Would You Do?* showed reactions of people in public towards an elderly person being harassed by teenagers. You might think that everyone came to the elderly person's aid, but sadly many walked by and ignored the teenagers' treatment of the old woman. What does that say about us as a society and about how we treat the elderly?

Our experiences influence the formation of our thoughts, words, and actions, whether we perceive them as good or bad. I would venture to guess the majority of us are outraged when we see an elderly person being beat up on the nightly news, whether our previous experiences with the elderly are good or bad. But how would you feel if you witnessed some form of disrespect that was much less violent? Physical abuse is much less prevalent than the blatant disregard and disrespect we have as a society towards aging adults, but the feelings that result from being disregarded and disrespected are much the same. Imagine that a man living in a long-term care facility is abruptly woken up, quickly pushed into going to the bathroom, literally pulled and tugged through getting dressed, and rushed to breakfast without getting his face washed or teeth brushed. The nurse's aide, who criticizes how long it takes to feed the residents, shoves food in his mouth while discussing her personal life with the other aides, without ever a kind word to the resident—day after day. Is the resident's feeling of worthlessness any different? Yet this happens every single day to thousands of seniors, and we allow it. We don't see that treatment as abuse.

Few of us seem able to put ourselves in the shoes of an aging adult, because our experience of aging and knowledge about the physical, psychological, and emotional changes that occur are far from our view, thoughts, and understanding. Our society sometimes ignores what we fear, and aging is something we fear. Most of us don't want to think about it, talk about it, or be involved with it, even though we know we'll most likely become old someday.

I want you to purposely take time to think about your own experiences and thoughts on aging before going on to the next chapter. As you continue reading, throughout this book, I want you to review your own thoughts and feelings as I take you deeper into the aging process, share real stories of seniors, and offer solutions to the problems we face together. Aging is not a segment of life, as you will see in the next chapters, and neither are the problems associated with aging.

Chapter 2
Transfigured in Time
Our exterior transfiguration

From moment to moment, everything is being transfigured. With each second, minute, hour, day, and year, everything is aging and transforming. We don't recognize moment-by-moment changes because they are so subtle. Our physical bodies began aging the moment we were conceived. We wear the years and experiences on our bodies and face. Whether we are twenty, forty, or eighty, we can look at our bodies and see effects of aging. Scars from skinned knees, stretch marks following a pregnancy, or crow's feet around our eyes all reflect years gone by. The loss of elasticity in our skin and the battle wounds of life leave additional and deeper impressions in our skin as we age. Our outside appearance shows physical evidence as we all watch how well or poorly we age, but the fact is that every blood vessel, brain cell, organ, and system is experiencing the slow subtle changes of aging just as our skin does. We are all aging.

Will you focus on the signs of aging with only a mirror view, or will you be introspective and see the grey hair and wrinkles as a by-product of what your life has evolved into from years gone by? Everything goes through metamorphosis, like a caterpillar to a gorgeous butterfly, or a bud to a beautiful rose, and you will too.

Seeing your first grey hair and wrinkles can cause fear and dread of aging, or you can view it as the unfolding of your life, like the rose that grows into the amazing fullness of what it can be. Although your exterior will be etched by your past, your soul never ages. Your soul is your past, present, and future. The essence of who you are internally is best described by a quote from Edward G. Bulwer-Lytton, "It is not by the grey of the hair that one knows the age of the heart."

It's very important to ask yourself what matters most. Be honest with yourself as you think about your inner and outer self. Are you the kind of person that will do everything possible to hang onto your youthful appearance, or are you more interested in working on the person you are on the inside?

I have had acquaintances in my life who have gone towards middle age kicking and screaming. One woman I recall, whom I knew through my kids' school, tried to hang onto youth so tightly she dressed too young, and she acted inappropriately and immature by intertwining herself with much younger people. She felt insecure and tried to find her worth in the flirtation with and response from much younger men. I felt bad for her. Her behavior and the way she dressed was a source of gossip in the community and took a toll on her marriage and relationships.

Who hasn't seen the women who have become so obsessed with retaining their youthful appearance that they've had so many plastic surgeries they have actually become plastic-looking and over-sculpted? Of course, these are extreme examples but not so uncommon. This is not to say we shouldn't try to look our best no matter what age we are. I just want to point out how much the fear of aging can cause such significant problems.

Unless the lady I used as an example comes to terms with the natural progression of aging, she will face even more difficulty later in life. She will also miss the beauty of the experience. I enjoy the wisdom I've gained over the years and the comfort of who I am, and I look forward to becoming an even better me. If we're so busy fighting against nature, we won't have the time to think about our place in this world and how to be our best selves.

Physical loss

Grey hair and wrinkles are only two of the many changes that occur, and can occur, with aging. In what shape would you find yourself if you lost your vision, hearing, sense of smell, taste, or touch after living a full life with everything intact? As our bodies age, we will most likely experience some loss. Whether we need reading glasses or become fully blind from macular degeneration, whether we suffer from a slight hearing loss or need hearing aids, we will have loss. We wear out our body parts like a car. Some of your parts will wear better than others, but you will wear out.

Genetics, environment, and self care-all play a role in how we age, but even those who had healthy parents, who lived in a clean and healthy environment and did everything possible to take care of their health can lose their health and mobility. Individuals who eat healthy diets, don't smoke or drink, manage stress well, exercise, and adhere to preventative health care guidelines wear out and can find themselves suffering from a life-altering disease or loss of mobility as they age. Following a healthy lifestyle reduces those chances, but nothing is guaranteed.

What emotions would you experience with a loss of your senses or the ability to walk? I think we go through life like teenagers, in a sense, believing we're invincible and thinking it won't happen to us. As much experience as I have with the elderly, and as much as I try to prepare for aging, even I have some difficulty seeing myself unable to walk or losing my hearing. I wonder more often whether I'll be able to remain independent or end up getting Alzheimer's than I do thinking about specific losses. I hope that I will handle any decline or significant changes in my senses or mobility well, but unless or until we actually experience those kinds of losses or changes, we won't know our reaction. Preparing our mind for the possibility will help us cope when our parts fail to serve us well.

There are more common losses related to aging than others. Most of us will lose some hearing ability, lose clarity of vision, and have a tougher time with mobility from arthritis as we age. The range of loss can be minor to total loss. Baby boomers, in particular, spent hours upon hours listening to blaring music that probably caused more hearing damage than in generations before us, but we won't feel the full effects until we are in our seventies and eighties. My husband started feeling the effects of hearing loss early in life from his previous work in loud factories. Vision loss is common beginning around forty. According to the Mayo Clinic, farsightedness as we age is the gradual loss of your eyes' ability to focus actively on nearby objects. It's a natural, often annoying part of aging that usually continues to worsen until around age sixty-five.

According to the Centers for Disease Control (CDC), fifty percent of adults age sixty-five and older report a diagnosis of arthritis, which is the most common cause of lost mobility, but arthritis isn't the most prevalent cause. One out of three seniors fall every year. More than two million seniors were treated in emergency rooms for injuries due to a fall in 2009. Twenty to thirty percent of people who fall suffer moderate to severe injuries such as lacerations, hip fractures, or head traumas. These injuries can make it hard to get around or live independently.

I have cared for many aging adults whose lives were totally changed by a fall. For example, my agency was called by a spouse to provide assistance to her husband after a fall that devastated their lives. This gentleman and his wife were visiting a local museum, and somehow he fell on the marble steps and hit his head so hard he suffered a closed-head injury that left him unable to care for himself. Prior to the fall, he was an extremely intelligent, active, prestigious private pilot. He had just purchased a new car and had no plans of slowing down. In an instant, everything changed. Whoever expects something like that to happen? A normal day just taking a trip to an art museum, and their whole lives changed. His memory was so affected that he could no longer be left alone. This injury not only affected him, it affected his wife, family, work, and friendships. This was one of the worst results of a fall I'd personally seen. I can't count the number of patients I've had who suffered lost mobility from fractures after a fall.

Imagine for a moment that you could no longer hear your spouse or children laughing. What about losing the ability to read or see anything clearly? What if your ankles, knees, and hips were so affected by arthritis, it was too painful to walk? What if you enjoyed cooking or writing, but your hands were so crippled by arthritis that holding anything small was impossible? These losses not only affect you physically, they affect how you function in the world and whether you can continue to do things you enjoy. They can affect your independence and self esteem.

How would you handle loss? Will you be angry or thankful that there is a device to compensate for the loss or an alternative way to function? Most types of loss can be accommodated in some form or another. Glasses are acceptable to most of us because they don't indicate only aging. Children, teens, and young adults wear glasses, so none of us think anything about an elderly person wearing glasses.

Hearing loss is another story. Most individuals with hearing loss do not wear hearing aids. The prevalence of hearing aids in completely deaf children or young adults is low; therefore, hearing loss is attached to aging in a stereotypical way. This stereotype causes seniors with hearing loss to be resistant to using a hearing aid, often leaving them excluded from socializing simply because they cannot hear the conversation. Feeling excluded can lead to additional problems, such as anger, isolation, and depression. Rather than accept the loss and use a hearing aid to stay engaged in life, many seniors are bothered by the negative perception.

Many mobility problems can be dealt with by using a cane, walker, or wheelchair. What's even more important is using those devices for preventing falls and injuries that will cause even more loss of mobility. There are two groups of people: the ones who accept their mobility limitations and easily adapt to using one type of equipment, and the others who refuse because they're in denial or they do not want to be seen using a cane, walker, or wheelchair.

My parents represent each end of the spectrum. My mom's mobility has been affected by a history of back surgeries, hip replacements, and a knee replacement. She will not go anywhere without her cane. She has no problem using the electric scooter when she goes shopping or finding out if a place or event she plans on going to can accommodate her needs. She accepted the loss and decided she will do what she must to remain mobile and active, without any regard for what people think. My dad's mobility has been affected by arthritis, neuropathy in his feet and legs, and knee replacements. He will not use a cane, walker, or motorized scooter. Instead, he limits his activity and refrains from going any place where too much walking is required. My dad is apparently more focused on people's perceptions of him than on being active, which saddens me. My mom is out and about, enjoying life, and my dad spends way too much time at home missing out.

Will you concentrate on living life or foregoing life because of the stereotypical perceptions of aging when you are faced with loss? What will you expect of yourself and those around you if you lose your vision, hearing, or mobility? Will you see yourself as less of a person, or will you still feel whole if your vision is gone one day, or you can no longer walk? These are real questions to ask yourself now so you can better prepare yourself for the future. Ignoring these real-life possibilities will only cause more difficulty for you when you are faced with loss. Denial and acceptance are distinguishable in how aging adults live their last decades. The example of my mom and dad shows how much their different perspectives affect their day-to-day life.

What constitutes a whole person? Do you think the loss would take away from the soul of who you are? Should you be treated differently, less respected, or less valued because of some natural or unavoidable loss? Loss is difficult in any form. We have all had loss: loss of a pet, a family member or friend, a job, or a relationship. But a physical loss of one or more of our senses is much different. It affects the way we perceive ourselves and how we function in the world. Some loss is gradual, some is sudden, but either way it is completely natural to need time to process the loss and grieve it. It is also absolutely necessary to accept it and adjust in order to continue living a full and happy life.

This is a great time to share my personal story of loss and how I have handled it, because it offers an example about loss and acceptance. In December 2003, just sixteen months after opening my homecare agency, I got extremely sick. I assumed I would see my doctor, have a diagnostic test or two, get a prescription for something, and be on my way. Little did I know I would spend the next five years so sick from a mystery illness I literally didn't know if I'd live or die. My life as I knew it was gone. I spent more time in bed during those five years than I care to think about. It was the first time in my life I needed help to do the basic things I'd always done, like clean my house or prepare myself a meal. At times, I needed someone to drive me to an appointment or pick me up from wherever I had driven when I realized I was too sick to drive myself home.

I had always been the caregiver, never the care receiver. I found losing independence to be very difficult, and I didn't ask for help unless it was absolutely necessary. Those five years brought a range of emotions including sadness, hope, loneliness, and mostly depression from losing my active, healthy life and being limited by my body. I could no longer do the physically active work I had done, and I spent lots of time thinking about the life I'd lost and the things I was no longer able to do.

Finally, after five years of doctors and more diagnostic tests and medications than I care to think about, I was diagnosed with chronic fatigue syndrome and Sjögren's syndrome, two chronic incurable illnesses. There I met the decision to either continue to grieve my once active, healthy life and remain miserable, or accept my new life with chronic illness, concentrate on what I could do, and live as happily as possible.

I decided to accept my new life. I thought about what I loved doing, which was helping seniors with education, information, and advocacy. I thought about what I may be able to do from home. You see, I wake up every single day in pain and feel like I have the flu. I take my medications and pray I can function physically. Some days I can and some days I can't, but even when I can, I have to limit my activity or I'll land myself back in bed.

Weighing my passion and focusing on what I was still able to do, I decided to write a blog. I thought that I could share the education, experience, knowledge, information, and resources I had shared in hospitals, rehabilitation centers, long term care, assisted living facilities, and homes from my laptop in bed. My initial goal was to help a few seniors and their families with information prior to unexpected illness or injury so their stress would be reduced when a crisis happened, and they would be better prepared to make informed, appropriate, and quick decisions.

My life quickly changed from depression and grief to excitement and happiness. Actually, I've never been happier! Although I had never thought about being a writer or helping people beyond my community, my articles quickly gained attention and things progressed from there.

The whole key to changing my life from misery to happiness was accepting my limitations and moving on with life despite the loss. Although I learned this lesson earlier in my life than I'd expected, or than I'm addressing in this book, the lesson is the same. Accepting and learning to live well in bodies that no longer do what they used to will be very important in living our aging years well. If I had continued to focus on what I couldn't do and what I physically lost, I would have never found the happiness I have now. I have gone to pain and illness support groups, chat rooms, groups on Facebook and groups on the internet. Very few have a positive tone. Most participants commiserate with each other, focusing on the problems and difficulties rather than how to live better and happily.

Do you think focusing on the negative aspects of loss are helpful or damaging? We've all heard that misery loves company. You will become what you focus on: miserable or fulfilled and happy. Can you see how much perspective means to our lives? Do you want to live a happy life despite the challenges and losses you'll face? Your perspective of yourself and your life determines how well or poorly you will age.

Our interior transfiguration

Our thoughts, personalities, and perspectives are also being transfigured as time goes by. We don't think of our thoughts or personalities as aging, but they are. What adult hasn't said, "If I only knew then what I know now?" Of course, we learn over time and that brings about changes in who we are, but I don't think we give enough credit to what experiences do to our thoughts, personalities, and perspectives.

One day, as I thought about wisdom and age, I started thinking about life as a mountain and us as the climbers. Each decade of life is another level on the mountain. As we make it to our twenties, thirties, and so on, we are only able to see as far as the level we have climbed. We cannot see further up the mountain because we haven't been there yet. We can only see where we've been. There are many different paths to each level, or decade of age, on the mountain so although we don't see or follow all the paths others have taken, we still make it to the next level. I picture this in my mind now as a fifty-year-old woman. I think back to when I hit the previous decades of my life and compare it to levels on the mountain. The level I'm currently on becomes a clearer picture of my life. When I was twenty years old, I only had the knowledge and experiences from the path I took to that level, my first nineteen years. I thought I had reached the thirty- or forty-year-old level of knowledge, as we all do when we're young. But I only had a very small view of the mountain. Now that I've crossed over the fifty-year mark, I have much more knowledge, experience, and perspective from the middle of the mountain than when I started.

No matter your age, you can understand that those who have lived longer and climbed to higher levels have a much bigger perspective. When I think of aging in those terms, it makes me want to learn more from those who have taken the paths that I'm about to embark on. As a society, we are not taking advantage of the knowledge, experience, and perspectives of those who have gone before us. Most of us can see how stupid that is when we think about it in terms of paths to a higher place on the mountain. Shouldn't we want to know how to avoid the difficulties, how to climb smarter and better, and what we may encounter on the way? All of that is available to us if we seek the knowledge and wisdom of the elderly.

I would guess, at this point, you are thinking it makes sense, yet most of society ignores the thoughts, opinions, and experiences of its elders, dismissing them as if they don't matter. We don't look at the beauty of our elders and what they have to offer. We have heard the saying, "Work smarter, not harder." Wouldn't you like to live smarter, not harder? We can avoid mistakes and struggles if we seek the advice and wise counsel from those who have gone before us. As long as we're alive, it's not too late to take advantage of learning and seeking the wisdom of our elders.

Aging is more than just broken bodies and wrinkled faces. A scripture in Proverbs says it all: "Young people take pride in their strength, but the grey hairs of wisdom are even more beautiful" (Prov. 20:29). If we think about the mountain again, from start to finish, it's easy to see how we all start energetic and physically strong with wonder and fearlessness. As we reach higher levels, the climb becomes physically more difficult, and we experience injuries, detours, and maybe some fear, but we must learn how to get through difficulties, solve problems, and work around our limitations to continue. We need to enjoy the journey and see the beauty in the climb. The beauty of the view is in our memories, lessons, knowledge, wisdom, and perspective.

Perspective from the top levels of the mountain and the decades as we age is very different from our perspective at the lower levels of the mountain in our younger years. We become more comfortable with ourselves, more assured, in many ways more peaceful and settled, but that is only if we didn't resist the difficulty of the climb. How high we make it on the mountain or how old we become is not ultimately in our control. If we resist going further because the climb becomes too difficult, or we don't enjoy the beauty, we waste our years dreading what's to come. If we see the difficulties as a challenge and overcome them, keep our goal in mind, and appreciate the beauty of the climb, we will enjoy our elder years. How we perceive life and deal with difficulties will have a lot to do with how we age. The old cliché, "Life is a journey, not a destination" is very important to understand. We should choose to have the greatest journey ever, not just a great journey until we reach retirement and then forget it all.

Some elders are completely at peace and comfortable with life, and others are miserable. We can't and won't ever know all the details of the paths of their lives, or if we might be given the same path, but we can seek the wisdom of our elders, try to understand life from their perspective, and ask their advice. If you opened a business for the first time and had to choose between winging it based on your own knowledge and experience or learning from someone who succeeded in the same business, what would you choose? Why should life be different? Life is much more important than a business venture.

Most seniors like to talk about their lives, experiences, and how they see the world, yet many are never asked. In preparing for this book, a couple of the people I interviewed became emotional just from being asked to be interviewed. That told me it has been awhile since they felt valued. Imagine if no one cared to get to know you. Imagine if your thoughts, opinions, and friendship didn't matter. There is nothing like seeing the sparkle in an elderly person's eyes as they talk about and relive the enjoyable and happy times in their younger years. You can almost see the video of their life playing in their minds through their eyes. If you haven't seen life through an elderly person's eyes, I highly suggest you do, because it is a very special experience.

Taking time to simply sit and talk with elderly people and to ask them about themselves and their lives can bring such happiness and joy, not only to them, but to you as well. I can honestly say my life has been enhanced by time spent with seniors, and your life can be too. If we are all climbing the same mountain on different paths, how can we not be interested in the experiences of others and in what's ahead? Don't we all want to avoid having our lives be more difficult than necessary? Wouldn't you like to know how to have the best experience possible and find the most happiness on the way? If you have children, you know that much of what you teach them is from experience so they don't have to learn the hard way and life is easier and happier than it was at times for you. Our elders are eager to do that for us if we just ask.

If you can keep the mountain in mind as you continue reading, you will get a clearer picture of how time transfigures us. The changes we experience physically, emotionally, and psychologically all come from our climb into our older years. Some of what happens to us is in part a result of our choices, and other things are beyond our control, just as any mountain climber could tell you. Our paths are very specific to us and our individuality, so understand that we all have a very unique perspective of ourselves, the elderly, and the world. Knowledge can and does change perspective. You will find this to be true from the perspective you had when you opened this book to the perspective you will have when you finish reading it. No matter what your background or experience is with the elderly, you will learn and understand more about aging by the time you finish this book.

The most difficult change of all

We have spent time thinking about our aging bodies, decline in abilities, and losing our senses, but those are all minor in comparison to losing our memories. Losing the very thing that makes us who we are is the greatest loss of all. Our entire identity in relation to ourselves and others resides in our memory. The childhood we had, the families we grew up with, the schools we went to, the people we married, the children and friends we have, the work we've done, and the emotions, values, and personality we developed are all contained in our memories. Listening to a siren that warns of an emergency involves memory. Using a toothbrush or a fork to eat dinner involves memory. Receiving and reciprocating love involves memory. We have memories that permit us to function on autopilot in our everyday worlds. We don't have to think that a glass is for drinking, or that our house is located on a certain road, or that the word *apple* represents a piece of fruit. We just know. We have experiential memories that we can use to recall joy, or sorrow, or how we developed feelings for someone. We have other memories that guide our thoughts and values, help us determine right from wrong, and allow us to distinguish loved ones from strangers.

Imagine if you slowly lost the ability to recall simple words that you knew your whole life. Sure, we have all experienced occasional times when a word doesn't come to us, but what about when a common word like house has no meaning? What would it be like for you to get in the car, intending to drive to the store only to find yourself in an unfamiliar place where you don't recognize anyone or anything, and you have no idea where to go or what to do? How frightening it must be to know you are losing your memories and there is nothing you can do to stop it. Losing the ability to recall your spouse or partner of fifty years is not only devastating to you, it is also devastating to your family and friends.

When I give the example of forgetting a partner or spouse of fifty years, it suggests that Alzheimer's is a disease that affects only individuals in their senior years. But, according to the Alzheimer's Association, Alzheimer's affects approximately ten percent of all cases of dementia in people who are in their forties and fifties. You may be reading this, imagining that you may only need assistance and care in old age, when it could be as soon as next year or the year after. Alzheimer's doesn't discriminate. It affects both men and women, and people of every race, socioeconomic background, and educational background in every part of the world.

As you continue to think about the mountain, think about memory loss. Dementia begins with short-term memory loss. It would be as if you remember beginning your climb on the mountain, but somewhere in the middle, you got lost. You can't remember how you got there, or why you are there. Initially, you would recognize that your memory is failing you. You would have days in which you remember more than other days, but as you continue the climb, you lose more memories of how you got where you are and what you're supposed to do there. You don't remember if you are supposed to go down, wait where you are, or go towards something. With progressive dementia, there would come a time when you would not even be aware that you have lost your memory, because you don't remember you ever had one. Your family and friends continue to grieve as they watch the person they know and love disappear.

I recently attended a family lunch gathering set up at a restaurant that included my mom, my aunts and uncles, a cousin, a second cousin, and my husband. We don't see each other often, so when we do it's usually a loud gab fest! One of my uncles has Alzheimer's. The last time I saw him was a few years ago before he had Alzheimer's. I don't know specifically how long it had been since others had seen him, but since they live much closer to each other I suspect they have seen him decline. He is in the severe stages of Alzheimer's; he can no longer carry on a conversation and his behavior is unrestrained. I had no problem interacting with him because of my education and experience, but that was not the case for others in my family.

My uncle was rather loud and made a lot of noises imitating cars, birds, and things like that. He was very joyful, but could not control his behavior, volume, or speech, and wasn't able to respond appropriately to conversation. Some members of my family were uncomfortable and didn't know how to respond, react, or interact with him, so they tried not to. I glanced around the restaurant at the looks on strangers' faces that seemed to express disgust and shock.

My husband cared for his parents who had Alzheimer's, so he completely understood, was at ease with my uncle, and related to him so that he would feel included and comfortable. On the ride home, I told my husband that it makes me sad that we have not come to a point in our society that the folks in this restaurant couldn't recognize that my uncle had Alzheimer's. People are still so uncomfortable being around someone who has this disease, they don't know how to interact. The lack of knowledge and understanding is prevalent in people who have no direct and regular contact with individuals suffering from this horrible disease, and the only thing that can improve that is by providing more education and exposure to affected persons.

We fear Alzheimer's. We dread hearing that diagnosis, and avoid those who often seclude themselves in shame, even though they have done nothing to bring that horrible disease upon themselves. We reject what we fear, and that is causing a delay in education, acceptance, understanding, and research. Our fear contributes to the shame, isolation, depression, and loneliness too often experience by people with Alzheimer's and other dementias, as well as their family caregivers. Shouldn't we embrace people who are losing their memories to help them enjoy as much of their life as they can? Shouldn't we embrace the spouses, sons, daughters, and other loving family and friends who give their time, love, and lives to care for loved ones who may one day not recognize who they are?

Maybe it will help to know that the memories are still deep within the mind. They aren't really lost. A disease has caused the inability to recall the memories. If you had Alzheimer's, you wouldn't really be gone. In the depths of dementia there can be lucid moments that prove the memories are there. People with Alzheimer's are trapped in a mind that no longer functions in a healthy, deliberate way. As horrifying as dementia is, having it can produce the most profound love anyone has ever been able to give. To unconditionally love, care for, and protect a spouse, parent, or friend with memory loss is a true and deep love. To fully give without expecting to receive anything is amazing and beautiful. A moment of lucidity can be appreciated as simply the connection of souls that has always been there.

I watched my aunt interact with my uncle at lunch. I was happy that she continues to include him and brought him with her; she didn't feel like she had to leave him with someone or hide him, and he was beyond feeling embarrassed or ashamed of his memory loss. She interacted with her husband by including him, attending to him, keeping calm when he became loud, and redirecting him as needed. She loves and remembers the man she married and didn't let this disease get in the way of that love. Seeing the unconditional love she has for him warmed my heart.

Imagine for a few minutes the fear of losing yourself and whether you have anyone in your life who has that kind of deep, unconditional love for you. Understand what individuals and families go through when they face and deal with Alzheimer's or other dementias. Could you expect that kind of love? Could you give deep and committed love without expecting anything in return?

From an empathetic perspective of early dementia, how do you think you'd handle the diagnosis? How would you handle informing family and friends? Would you work at being educated, work on a plan with your family and try to enjoy every single memory, or would you withdraw, deny the love of family and friends, and lose the last chance of remembering a good life and creating lasting memories for your family and friends?

Every year in mid November, the Alzheimer's Foundation of America (AFA) sponsors National Memory Screening Day. Thousands of participants all over the country partner with the AFA to offer screenings, educational programs, and support for individuals concerned about or dealing with memory loss. Early diagnosis is critical for early treatment, education, and planning for a better quality of life. The AFA's goal is to help individuals get diagnosed earlier so patients have a better chance of possibly delaying progression of the disease with early intervention. Early education better prepares patients and families to accept the truth of Alzheimer's and all that comes with the diagnosis. The National Memory Screening Day can be helpful to those concerned with or dealing with memory loss or Alzheimer's. Many people don't know there are other causes of dementia, and some of those are reversible. Reducing ignorance benefits everyone in our society.

In 2010, we offered the memory screening at my office for the first time. The AFA provided educational materials and resources to make available to participants. In addition, we offered two presentations on communicating with someone who has Alzheimer's. Knowing how to communicate is necessary in reducing stress, frustration, and anger when providing care. We purchased beverages, a variety of fruit, pastries, cookies, and snacks for the event, and we spent a lot of time preparing and promoting the event. Not one person came to receive a memory screening, view the presentation, get educational materials, ask questions, or receive support.

A nurse friend of mine who owns a homecare agency just over an hour away also offered the memory screen that day. She also did not have one participant. In a way, I was relieved that it wasn't my lack of preparation that resulted in zero participants. But it did cause me to wonder why and to wonder how many other sites across the nation had the same experience.

The AFA quickly followed up to inquire how the event went and what was the turnout. Needless to say, there wasn't much I could contribute to their survey. I concluded this experience by writing an article for *The Alzheimer's Reading Room* titled, "The Fear, Stigma, and Shame of Alzheimer's Disease," because I believe fear was the primary reason we didn't have any participants. We avoid what we fear. We fear the word *Alzheimer's* and dread that diagnosis. Those who receive the diagnosis of Alzheimer's disease often feel shame and isolate themselves from family and friends, declining even quicker because the isolation and shame are followed by depression and loss of socialization and activities, which then causes more stress on the psychological and emotional health of the individual.

Fear and denial are damaging to the person affected by memory loss. I have met many families in denial. Just recently, I dealt with an irate son who was angry that I suggested a geriatric evaluation for his mom due to her recent memory loss and paranoia. He proceeded to tell me that he knew all about senior health because he was an attorney and *guardian ad litem* for other seniors, and there was nothing wrong with his mother. His denial is causing his mother to live an anxious and fearful life because he refuses to have her evaluated and treated. Allowing someone to be tormented by their own thoughts, delusions, or hallucinations because you can't accept the truth boarders on neglect and abuse, as far as I'm concerned. People who deny the possibility of Alzheimer's or other dementias in a loved one are concerned only with their own feelings of fear and loss and are not focusing on doing the best for their loved one's peace and comfort.

There would never be that kind of fear regarding a health screening that included blood pressure checks, blood sugar checks, or other assessments of physical health issues. Why do we not look at mental health diseases as physical diseases of the brain, as diabetes is a disease of the pancreas or lupus is a disease of the immune system? Why is the thought process about brain diseases so obviously different?

Patients can do many things to prevent diabetes, but there are no reliable ways to preventing Alzheimer's, schizophrenia, or clinical depression. These are diseases that can affect anyone without provocation. They can affect you, me, and anyone we love and care for, yet we fear them, we don't want to be around people who have them, we don't want to talk about them, and if one of them should strike us, we want to hide in shame, fear, and embarrassment. Somehow, some way, we need to change our way of thinking about brain diseases and the people affected.

Even the term mental health needs to be changed, because as long as I've known, just the term *mental health* conjures up fear and stigma. I wonder if our thinking would change if we called these illnesses *brain diseases*. Ask yourself if that makes a difference, and if it does, change your own language. Since the perception and stigma have come from a very long history of ignorance, it will require a change in us all to remove the fear, stigma, and shame associated with brain diseases.

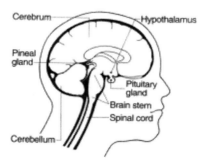

I am still wondering why no one came to the educational presentations we offered on Memory Screening Day. That part of the event was geared towards family caregivers of those already diagnosed. Was it partly an attempt to keep their loved one's illness private? Was it because they didn't want to be in a room with reminders of Alzheimer's disease? Was it because family caregivers thought it was nothing new, that they'd heard it all before? I guess I'll never know. I decided not to offer the memory screening again as a formal event. I will continue to educate, advocate, and support people and families affected by Alzheimer's disease and other dementias as well as care providers in other ways. I will refer those who have concerns of memory loss to specialists who can appropriately diagnose, but I will not offer it as a public event again.

How would you feel if you were diagnosed while the stigma remains? Should you have to withdraw from your life in shame because we don't understand? What would it feel like to you if people stared, whispered, laughed, or insulted you because a disease took your memory and inhibitions? If you find the thought as sad as I do, what will you do differently from now on? Will you advocate, educate, correct a misinformed friend, or pull a child or teen aside who is acting out of ignorance to explain to them the terrible effects of Alzheimer's? Whether you are a medical professional, healthcare worker, family caregiver or not, once you know the truth you can help remove the stigma.

Who is affected by Alzheimer's?

Unless a treatment or cure is found soon, I expect that every single one of us will be directly affected by Alzheimer's and other dementias in one way or another. According to the Alzheimer's Association's 2011 Facts and Figures Report (http://www.alz.org/downloads/Facts_Figures_2011.pdf), an estimated 5.4 million people have Alzheimer's disease now. This doesn't take into account those living with memory loss who have yet to seek a full evaluation and diagnosis. I have met many in my own community.

Economic figures from the AFA's 2011 report reveal that Alzheimer's currently costs $183 billion a year. Yes, BILLION! If you don't think that affects you, think again. Sadly, more people take note when something as devastating as Alzheimer's disease affects the economy. The 183 billion does not take into account the unpaid care that family members are providing, which the Alzheimer's Association estimates to be valued at over 200 billion.

Currently, someone develops Alzheimer's every sixty-nine seconds—basically one person every minute. It is estimated that by mid century, one person will develop Alzheimer's every thirty-three seconds, almost double the current rate. Two people will develop Alzheimer's every minute. If we look at the current figure of $183 billion a year in costs, the projected increase will be estimated at $1.1 trillion by 2050. Anyone under the age of sixty reading this book can surely expect to be alive in 2050, especially since we are living increasingly longer.

What do you think your chances are of being one of the people who develops Alzheimer's in any given minute on any day? Current statistics reveal that one person in eight has Alzheimer's or another type of dementia. By mid century, the prevalence will increase to one person in four. What does that say about your chances of developing life-altering memory loss? If you sat at a dinner table with seven friends today, one of you can expect to lose the memories of your life.

Whether it is you or one of your friends who develops the disease, are you prepared? Is there someone to care for you or can you truthfully say you will care for your friend? How will you expect to be treated? How will you live? Where will you live? Will you want someone to advocate for you or your friend? This is the reality for someone every sixty-nine seconds right now, right here. My intent is not to scare you but to make you think and act. Ignoring the reality of the situation doesn't make it go away. It only makes you less prepared for a future crisis that in some way you will be affected by, either directly or indirectly.

Chapter 3
The Big Transition

Our lives go through marked transitional periods. We transition from babies to toddlers, to grade school children, to junior high and high school students, and into adulthood. Even though we go through changes in our thirties, forties, and fifties, there is no marked transition through our adult lives until we hit retirement.

When I think about transitions, the three that stand out as the biggest are puberty, becoming an adult on our own, and retirement. Thank God we know more at our retirement age than we did entering the other two periods, or I'm not sure we'd survive it! I'm not sure about you, but I would never want to go through puberty again! I wouldn't even want to start over as a young adult leaving my parents home.

The transition from busy days of work and raising children to retirement might be compared to going from your teen years to moving away from home and beginning your life as an adult, only it will be met with an enormous amount of reflection, which wasn't so much the case when we became adults, partly because we didn't have much to reflect on. If we think about the mountain again, when we enter our adult years, we are about one-fourth of the way up the mountain, and retirement is typically more like three-fourths of the way, give or take a few years. We have more to reflect on, more wisdom, and more experience behind us when retirement comes.

Depending on your age when you read this book, you will have different thoughts about retirement. If you are in your twenties, it probably seems a lifetime away. If you are middle aged, you are beginning to think about retirement and how close it is or you wish it was, depending on your financial status and whether you like the work you do. If you are retired, you have passed the threshold and may or may not be having difficulty with the transition.

I will celebrate my fifty-second birthday this year. I have never had a problem with aging, and turning fifty was great, but approaching my fifty-second year is causing me to stop and think about turning sixty. Yes, it's more than eight years away, but it seems so close. I don't have any fears about it, I just think about how much longer I may have to accomplish things that are important to me. Middle age brings about a deeper thought process about what we've done and what we will do with the time left. We even wonder how much time we may have left. Believe me when I tell you, if you're not there yet, the years go by very fast!

Time, energy, and socialization

We never felt there were enough hours when our days were filled with work, raising families, maintaining our daily lives, and the activities we were involved in. We seemed to have endless energy when we were young and did it all, but as the years pass our energy reserves decrease. When you were young, did you have no problem meeting friends at 11:00 p.m. because you had the energy to do so? As we age, we begin planning our time and energy more carefully. Friends we used to meet any night of the week at 11:00 p.m. become friends we meet on a weekend for an early dinner. We have some loss of social connection and begin focusing on using the energy we have to take care of the things we need to take care of. Activities are lost because we no longer have the energy to do them.

There are many losses and changes we will face when we retire. We lose the daily interaction and socialization with our co-workers or staff. Many of us will decide to downsize our home or move to another location. Couples can begin having problems when they start spending so much time together or a retiring spouse wants to move and the stay-at-home spouse doesn't want to leave familiar surroundings and friends.

If you have activities you love, such as golf, gardening, or volunteering and you no longer have the energy to do them, how will you feel? I recently started thinking about amusement parks and roller coasters. I love roller coasters but haven't been on one for a few years now. I thought about riding a roller coaster again, but I didn't know if I would have the energy to walk for hours in the heat and stand in the lines. I wondered if my body could handle being whirled in an upside down position anymore. I wondered if I had already ridden a roller coaster for the last time.

Recently, my husband and I went on vacation to visit my brother, Joe, who lives near Orlando, Florida, which is an amusement-park haven. My brother and I rode many roller coasters together since we were kids, and had lots of fun doing it! Since we still love to have fun together like when we were kids, we went to Sea World. Sea World added roller coasters since I was there many years ago. The experience was different than the last time I rode a rollercoaster. My brother, my husband, and I are older now, so our pace was more leisurely. We didn't hurry from one ride to another. We agreed there would be no way we'd wait for hours in line like we did when we were kids. But we enjoyed the day just as much. As far as the actual roller coaster ride . . . well, I think my days of being upside down on a ride are over. The ups and downs of the ride were great, but the inversion of the loop-the-loops were a bit much for my stomach. It didn't bother my husband or brother, and after a couple rides I was perfectly fine relaxing on the bench while they rode again. I'm glad I went for it and don't have to wonder if I missed knowing whether I'd ever ride again. I will choose carefully when the opportunity comes in the future, and I'm completely fine with giving up the full-body inversion I once loved so much.

Do you wonder how long you'll be able to do and enjoy activities as you age? Will you use the opportunities that come to you or make your own opportunities to enjoy whatever you can? Some activities will be lost without your realizing they are gone, others will be lost suddenly by an injury or illness that won't allow you to return to that activity again. Some activities you'll give up because you lack interest or lose the energy or stamina required to do them. According to a 2008 National Institute on Aging report, the proportion of leisure time that older Americans spend socializing and communicating—such as visiting friends or attending social events—declines with increasing age from thirteen percent for ages fifty-five to sixty-four to ten percent for ages seventy-five and over. The proportion of leisure time devoted to sports, exercise, recreation, and travel also declines with age. On an average day, most Americans age sixty-five and older spend at least half of their leisure time watching television. Americans age seventy-five and older spend a higher proportion of their leisure time reading, relaxing, and thinking than did those ages fifty-five to sixty-four. Yet, a study published February 13, 2012 in the *Journal of Aging Research* found that healthy older adults reported less negative thinking compared to other age groups, leading to greater life satisfaction in seniors.

When activities and socialization are lost, what will bring you joy? What will fill your days? What will you have the energy to do? Will you find joy in a meal? Will your big activity of the week be a doctor appointment? Will you be satisfied with how you spend your time, or will you have regrets? I don't want to waste life or end up in a state of regret.

Economic transition

Our financial status now determines our retirement age more than ever before. Historically, we were secure in working a job for thirty or more years and then retiring at age sixty-five with a comfortable pension. This is no longer the case. Recent changes in job stability, corporate corruption, and poor management of government dollars has left retirees without the pensions they earned and counted on. Employees feel less protected by and loyal to a specific company. All of us wonder if Social Security will exist in the next few years. Retirement security from years of dedication to an employer are gone.

Whether we have the money to retire at sixty-five or not, we will still experience economic changes when we do retire, unless we are in the extremely small percentage of individuals who are beyond what any average person would consider wealthy. We must think about our retirement income in terms of the number of years we expect to live, especially if we plan on living on our retirement savings, which is quickly becoming the norm. I think most of us recognize that pension plans will soon be a thing of the past. Many people who have lived and worked under the assumption that their pension would be there for them have found themselves out in the cold. Not knowing the number of years we will live, it's very difficult to budget retirement money through the remainder of one's life. I have met many people who were running out of money, or feared they would, because they were living longer than they expected or needed to spend more money on healthcare sooner than they expected.

We have all seen retirees greeting customers at Walmart or picking up part time jobs in other retail stores or businesses. Some are working because they like to get out and enjoy the social interaction, but I am sure more are there to earn additional money to support their lifestyle or pay for basic needs.

We can experience many losses due to a post-retirement decrease in income, from the home we live in, to the activities we participate in, to the friends we keep. If there is now a big discrepancy in your income and that of a friend whom you spent time with while you were working, you may not be able to maintain the same lifestyle and activities, and the friendship may grow apart. In our younger years, many of us experienced feeling excluded from activities with friends because our income didn't allow us to go out and do what they were doing. Or, our friends couldn't do the things we were able to do because their income was less than ours. In retirement, it is often the same.

I have come to believe, based on my personal observation, couples who have been together most of their adult lives and both had a career have more retirement income than a single person or a couple who married later in life. They generally have their house paid off and enjoy the typical comforts of life, so they will have more expendable income in their retirement years. People who divorced at forty usually find that they are starting over, don't have a home that's paid for, and may need to replace things lost in the divorce. Of course, this isn't always the case, but it would stand to reason that one person who lived on a more level playing field with a friend while they were working may end up parting ways because of income levels post retirement.

When I was young, my grandparents seemed fairly well off. Not rich by any measure, they had a beautiful home, my grandma shopped in higher-priced stores, and they appeared to be pretty comfortable. My grandfather retired from General Motors with a decent pension. Back in those days, spouses weren't automatically included in the pension. The employee had to elect to add them. My grandfather died in his mid seventies. I witnessed a quick and significant change in my grandmother's lifestyle. Years later, I learned that when she and my grandfather discussed adding her to the pension, she told him not to worry about it, that she would die before he did. She spent more than twenty years after his death struggling to make ends meet. They didn't think through the implications of their decision.

Many people give up things they enjoyed during their working life, such as travel or expensive hobbies like golf, because they can no longer afford them. When we're working, most of us can acquire extra income for vacations or activities through overtime pay, freelance work, or side jobs. If we work hard enough, we can find the money to do those things. This isn't so easy in our older years. Many employers prefer younger workers, making it more difficult for seniors to find employment.

The good news is that we tend to be more satisfied with life as we grow older. We focus more on what is important in life. Maintaining our health, family, relationships, and finding the simple joys in life are less expensive than acquiring the big house, fancy cars, and all the material things we wanted when we were young. There is a special peace that comes with that as long as we are not struggling and our health isn't failing.

Your retirement

Will you enter your retirement years with regret or acceptance? Imagine you are sixty-five and it's your retirement day, and then ask yourself these questions: Did you do enough, accomplish enough, and raise your children well enough? Did you follow your dreams or did you allow life to get in the way of what was really important to you, your happiness, and the happiness of your loved ones? Were you so wrapped up in work and raising children that now you don't know who you are without the work and kids? Or, will you be self-accepting? Will you feel like you lived the best life you could? Will you feel like you were aware of what was important? Will you be able to appreciate the joys and blessings, and the lessons from the difficulties you've faced? Will you feel satisfied and ready to accept the new phase in your life?

Essentially, we will all go from doing to being. How we perceive being is the difference between a successful or unsuccessful transition into our senior years. Although roles are changing, many women experience a loss of identity when the nest empties, and men can find themselves feeling less valued when the work they did has ended. We tend to find value in what we do rather than who we are.

Remember the feelings of satisfaction you had when you first helped a parent or a teacher when you were four or five years old? Those feelings of satisfaction can be renewed by service in your retirement years. What we seek is the feeling of being valued. Lying on the grass watching the clouds or running to the window to see a robin probably brought you joy and peace when you were a child. Are you bypassing the simple pleasures in the rat race of life? Will you renew those experiences when the constant pace of doing is over and you enter the world of being? Your perspective of what's important and what gives you joy is up to you as you age. You can embrace your elderly years or fear what's to come. Imagine for a moment, just being. Can you? Will you embrace a simpler life or be bored by it? Depending on your health and financial status, you may not have a choice. Loss of health and income can force you into a less active and simpler life whether you like it or not.

Our fears of aging vary around the globe, according to the Aging Services of California. In an international survey, the Dutch reported fearing weight gain, Germans reported worry about loss of eyesight and mental alertness, Belgians reported worry about incontinence, and Indians reported worries about getting grey hair or losing their hair all together. The MetLife Foundation reported that Americans fear Alzheimer's more than diabetes, heart disease, or stroke. Although the specific fears vary in different cultures, we can agree that there is a universal fear of aging.

Spirituality in aging

Spirituality is becoming more accepted and increasingly included in healthcare as studies show evidence of how our beliefs are connected to healing and aging. A 2006 study in *The Journal of Religion and Health* reported that spirituality and private religiosity contribute to higher physical well-being among older adults.

An article by the University of Maryland Medical Center titled, "Spirituality," offers a bit of the history of spirituality in healthcare and the influences of spirituality on health. The article states:

In most healing traditions and through generations of healers in the early beginnings of Western medicine, concerns of the body and spirit were intertwined. But with the coming of the scientific revolution and the enlightenment, these considerations were removed from the medical system. Today, however, a growing number of studies reveal that spirituality may play a bigger role in the healing process than the medical community previously thought.

Spiritual practices tend to improve coping skills and social support, foster feelings of optimism and hope, promote healthy behavior, reduce feelings of depression and anxiety, and encourage a sense of relaxation. By alleviating stressful feelings and promoting healing ones, spirituality can positively influence immune, cardiovascular (heart and blood vessels), hormonal, and nervous systems.

We cannot discount how much our spiritual beliefs play into how well we cope with aging and the health challenges we face. I know personally that

I would never have been able to get through everything I have since I lost my health without hope and my faith in God. I cannot separate my faith and beliefs from my life and well being, because they are who I am. My health is not separate. The medical community has professed that they have seen healing miracles that cannot be explained by medical science. We must address the whole person in aging and health. We do a disservice to the well-being of seniors everywhere if we don't ask about and include spiritual provisions in healthcare and long-term care. We don't have to believe or adhere to anyone else's beliefs, we just need to recognize and support the role of spirituality in senior living, health, and care.

Fear of aging

What is your fear? Is Alzheimer's your greatest fear? If we have witnessed a family member lose their life to this dreadful disease, we have seen that the losses are enormous. Losing the ability to direct one's own life is devastating. Your sense of security and destiny is in the hands of those who will provide your care. If you have Alzheimer's and you have a spouse, adult child, or family who will do everything possible to keep you home, loved, and safe, the devastation will not be as bad. But what if you don't? What if your family is not able to care for you, or you have no one? You will be facing a life without choices. Your surroundings will be based on your income and the decor chosen by the facility's owner, which may or may not be to your liking. Your meals, showers, activities, and care will all depend on the care providers' watch. You will not have a voice in your own life. If you've been to a nursing home or assisted living facility, what did you think? Are you okay with handing your life over to any of the care providers you've seen or known in a long-term care facility?

My friend Kathy Bradway, who owns Periwinkle Designs in Davison,

Michigan, is focused on changing the decor in long-term care facilities. She recently told me that when she asks families what they think of the decor, she often hears, "It's nice." She then poses the question, "Nice for whom? Nice for you?" Kathy said they often come back with, "Well, it's nice for my mom." Why do families think a facility is nice enough for a loved one when they wouldn't want to live there?

Would you want to live in or receive care in any of the long-term care facilities you've been to or have seen on TV or videos? Personally, I have no plans for living in a nursing home and will do whatever it takes now so that I don't end up there later! It's not that I don't think there are great care providers or nice facilities, but this is not where I want to spend my final years. I like my privacy, comforts of home, and the ability to adhere to my own schedule. I want my family to be comfortable spending time with me and not to be kept away by a dislike of nursing homes.

That said, we have heard the horror stories on the news. You can search "elder abuse" or "nursing home abuse" on YouTube and find video after video of very disturbing and sad stories. A couple months ago, there was a horrific finding in two different nursing homes in Michigan; one of the homes was in my community. In both nursing homes, patients were infested with maggots due to negligent care. One patient had a tracheotomy and was discovered to have an infestation of maggots in her neck. The other had a catheter, and maggots had infested her genital area. I hope that angers you as much as it did me! I publicly spoke out in response to the local news article and was subsequently contacted for an interview for a follow-up article. It's crazy to me that there is more public outrage and response to a neglected animal than there was to this news story! What kind of society have we become that we allow these things to happen and don't speak out? To my knowledge, I was the only person who professionally cares for seniors in my community who publicly spoke out about this.

I'm not sure what to conclude about that; I feel nothing other than total sadness. That no one else was willing to put their name on a public statement is a shame, a real shame.

What kind of people allow such horrific neglect? These are not isolated incidents. Good grief, this happened at two different nursing homes in two different cities! These weren't singled-out patients who were the only victims of neglect. Everyone who lives in these facilities is being neglected in one form or another. As I told the news reporter, this didn't just happen and it won't stop either. This poor treatment and care begins with the owner and spreads downward through the staff. Owners and administrators set the tone for care. Kind, compassionate, caring, ethical people who own and operate facilities or agencies make sure their staff provides the quality care they expect. If an owner is only in it for the money, they won't care about whom they hire or the people entrusted to their care

As we face enormous aging-population growth, more and more people are getting into senior care expecting to get rich off the baby boomers without any real concern for how they provide care or the people they will affect, and that is very frightening. Elder abuse is a growing problem and will continue to grow as people try to take advantage of the aging population. The National Center on Elder Abuse estimates 700,000 to 3.5 million seniors are abused, neglected, or exploited each year. The actual numbers are difficult to pin down because elder abuse is underreported and under-identified. According to the NCEA, as few as one in six cases are reported. The 2010 National Elder Mistreatment Study published in the American Journal of Public Health (vol. 100; pp. 292–297) indicated that approximately eleven percent of the 5,777 U.S. elders surveyed had experienced some type of abuse or potential neglect during the previous year. It is important to note that this survey did not include elders with dementia, a segment of the population believed to be at even greater risk for mistreatment, or elders living in long-term care facilities. As the aging population grows and more are diagnosed with Alzheimer's or other types of dementia, the incidences will increase without our ability to obtain the true numbers of abuse and neglect cases.

Although abuse may be perceived as physical or psychological battering, the most prominent form of abuse is neglect. Seniors are also suffering sexual abuse, and the rate of financial abuse and exploitation is increasing. According to a 2009 report by Met Life, seniors are losing a minimum of $2.6 billion annually as a result of financial abuse and exploitation. Elder abuse is recognized in the U.S. as a form of abuse, neglect, or exploitation at the hands of a trusted caregiver, so these estimates are not in relation to strangers abusing the elderly.

I have witnessed and worked with seniors and families who have been the victims of abuse. I have also reported incidences of abuse and neglect. I witnessed a woman being taken from her assisted-living home, screaming and crying, as her family put her in a less costly nursing home so they could preserve their inheritance. In another incident, after several months of attending to a homecare patient, I was told by the elderly woman that her daughter, with whom she lived, hit, screamed, neglected, and degraded her. I filed a report to Adult Protective Services, which I never made lightly. APS did an investigation and closed the case, because the senior woman did not want to move to a nursing home and so she minimized the extent of the abuse she had reported to me. This is often the case when an elderly person is subject to abuse by the family member that lives in the home with the patient. Living with abuse in their familiar home is preferred over living in an unfamiliar nursing home.

I met a woman who became a friend after she contacted me on a web site regarding financial abuse of her mother. Her brother was appointed the Power of Attorney over her mother's financial affairs. Her brother failed to pay his mother's assisted-living facility rent and healthcare policy premiums, and he spent the money she had in savings. My friend found out only after her mother, who has dementia, was being evicted from the assisted-living facility for nonpayment. They have lived a nightmare since. Her mother is now in a terrible nursing home that has neglected her, denied responsibility in physical injuries, and is nowhere close to the standard of care she was receiving at the assisted-living facility. My friend, who lives a long distance away and is chronically sick herself, is trying to lawfully make her brother accountable for her mother's financial loss and responsible to attend to their mother's care. And, she is now working as an advocate because of the brick walls she has hit with the legal system. Sadly and tragically, this is too often the case.

Beyond the discussion of the risk of abuse and neglect, do you think our eldercare system is sufficient or do you think there needs to be a change? There are many formidable factors that go into elder living and care. Must you live in a dingy nursing home with substandard care from untrained individuals because you don't have the money to live in a place that looks nice and has better care? Do you think your ability to pay should be the primary determinant of your life? In this current economic climate, we know that our financial situations can easily change. There are factors to consider. Whether you have a loved one who can provide care if you need it will play into your ability to afford professional care as you age. Many elderly individuals who worked hard, saved their money, and walked into retirement feeling comfortable have outlived their savings or had a crisis that devastated them financially. How many people have lost their retirement savings in the stock market or bad investments? Many of us assumed we would have real estate equity to draw from if we needed the money in retirement, and we all know how well that's going.

Both nursing homes cited above accept Medicaid for patients who can't afford to pay out of pocket for care. These poor people don't deserve to live like this just because they can't afford to pay for care, but they don't have the same options as people who can afford to pay. As far as I know, the patients are still in those facilities. If they don't have family support or the means to move to a better place, they are stuck. I offered my agency's services to anyone who wanted to move from one of the nursing homes and was contacted by one family. They reported that their dad was physically abused in that nursing home, but they didn't know of a good place he could move to that accepted Medicaid. All the places they knew of had waiting lists. I advised them of the places I know that are good and accept Medicaid, and some additional resources that could help. I have not heard from them since, so I hope they were able to move their father out of those deplorable conditions.

Although this picture is pretty grim from anyone's standpoint, we can make changes and provide better solutions for elder living and care. Think about what you want for yourself in your aging years. What do you want to see changed? What are you willing to do to bring about those changes?

Chapter 4
The Reality of Now
Current and future demographics

A week doesn't go by that we don't hear something on the news or see an article somewhere about baby boomers. As a baby boomer, I don't recall ever hearing about our generation with such focus and frequency. Why now? Because we are becoming seniors, and that is causing fear.

Before we go further let me just define baby boomer. The U.S. Census Bureau considers a baby boomer to be someone born between 1946 and 1964. The term was coined by Landon Jones in his book *Great Expectations: America and the Baby Boom Generation.* Seventy-six million Americans were born during those eighteen years, but the boom did not occur only in the U.S. The United Kingdom, Canada, Australia, and other allied countries also experienced this post-World War II population explosion. No generation before had such a large and steady population growth. Prior to 1946, the highest number of recorded births in a single year in the U.S. was 2.9 million births. The total number of births per year during the baby-boomer years ranged from 3.5 million to 4.3 million.

The U.S. Census Bureau reported the total U.S. population was 308,745,538 in 2010. Over 5.5 million persons—one in nine—were sixty-five years or older. One in five will be sixty-five years or older by the year 2035, nearly double the current senior population. During the next nineteen years, more than ten thousand baby boomers will turn sixty-five every day.

A good percentage of us baby boomers had half as many children as our parents did. As an example, my parents had four children who are now adults and can assist in their care. I have two adult children who may assist me. If one becomes ill or is financially unable to take time off work, the burden shifts from both to one adult child. Due to our current economic climate and the financial instability of Social Security, my sons may need to work far beyond what is considered normal retirement age, and perhaps no one will be available to assist me. Truthfully, I don't want to burden my sons with my care or count on them for my future needs. I must act now to secure my future care, and so should you.

Housing

There is evidence that there will not be enough long-term care facilities to house even a fair portion of the seventy-six million baby boomers who started turning sixty-five in January 2011. The Centers for Disease Control report, "Health, United States, 2010," states there were 15,700 nursing homes with 1,705,808 beds in the U.S. in 2009 (http://www.cdc.gov/nchs/data/hus/hus10.pdf#117). That's about one bed for every three people. That doesn't seem so bad, since we may expect that at least two out of three seniors will be healthy enough not to need nursing home services. But it's all changing, and quickly!

With the current instability of the economy and the possible end of Social Security, it is up to us now to secure our own retirements to the best of our abilities. More than any generation before us, those of us in our middle-age years feel increasingly fearful about how those years will be funded. Although people in their teens, twenties, and thirties don't think much about retirement, their financial planning should have already begun, because the longer they wait to invest in their retirement, the more difficult it will become to secure it.

MetLife provides some of the best and most up-to-date reports on aging and related issues. Their "2011 Market Survey of Long-Term Care Costs" reports that annual care costs currently range from $18,200 for adult day services to $87,235 for a private room in a nursing home. Fifteen percent of our current U.S. population is considered poor. I have had financial struggles, and at times I could not imagine paying $18,000 a year in living expenses, let alone spending that much for covering one third of my day. Adult day services are typically six to eight hours a day, five days a week; realistically, that isn't even one third of our week. The cost of assisted living currently averages over $41,000 a year. Genworth offers a care cost calculator based on individual states and types of living and care. The 4 types of care listed are homecare, adult day care, assisted living, and nursing home care. http://www.genworth.com/content/non_navigable/ corporate/about_genworth/industry_expertise/cost_of_care.html The calculator allows you to see current average costs and anticipated costs in the future for when you think you may need care. I currently live in Michigan. Average nursing home costs in Michigan for a semi private room in 2012 are over $80,000.00 per year. The calculator asks you "How long before you think you need care?" You can choose from a range of 10 years to 30 years from a drop down menu. I selected 20 years. The expected average costs in 2032 will be over $213,000.00! So if my husband and I actually need care in 20 years we are looking at nearly ½ a million dollars a year to live in a nursing home! Can you afford your future care? The only way I can see us affording care is by some financial miracle or a multi-million dollar win in the lottery. Don't you think we have to come up with an alternative for our future?

The breakdown of long-term care options

Unless you have researched eldercare for a family member or worked in the field, you may have some misconceptions about the different types of care or living arrangements available and what is covered by Medicare, Medicaid/MediCal, or health care insurance.

Long-term care falls into three basic categories: day care, residential care, and home care. The summary below describes the most typical living and care options currently available. New care models are being developed and tested across the country as we search for ways to care for the aging population and cut costs, but none have made a big enough mark to be among the most utilized yet.

Day care -

Day care - Day care is a program outside the person's residence they can attend and be monitored for typically six to eight hours daily. Most day-care programs are closed on weekends. These programs, even specialized memory day-care programs, have restrictions. While there is some variation in restrictions from program to program, they typically don't accept people with incontinence or people requiring medical attention other than giving oral medications and will not accept or tolerate people with any behavioral problems.

Residential care -

Rehabilitation - Rehab is temporary residential care with the goal of improving health and mobility, and is usually in a segmented area of a long-term skilled nursing facility. Medicare Part A covers 100% of the cost for twenty days if the patient has been hospitalized for a minimum of three days, not including the day of discharge. An inpatient stay doesn't begin when you enter the hospital, it begins when the doctor officially admits you to the hospital. You could be in the emergency department for hours, a holding room for another few hours and not actually be admitted for a day, so it's necessary to know whether you are an outpatient or inpatient to begin the three-day count. These policies have caused many folks to get a whopping bill they were unprepared for when they were discharged to a rehabilitation facility without meeting the three-day requirement.

With Medicare, you will be responsible to pay $141.50 for days 21-100, and you are responsible for 100% from day 101 on. Depending on the facility, but more likely than not, you will reside in a semi-private room. You receive meals, nursing care, assistance from a nurse's aide, physical and occupational therapy, possibly speech therapy if needed, and social work services. You will be seen and monitored by the facility physicians who provide the orders for your healthcare while you reside in the facility. Medications and any treatments or necessary equipment are provided under your insurance plan or are billed to you. Some equipment, such as walkers and wheelchairs, is owned by the facility; you have access to use that equipment during your stay but are responsible for your own once you leave the facility. Depending on the equipment you need, you may or may not have to pay out of pocket. Facilities, more often than not, will refer you to the companies they utilize without notifying you that you have the right to choose your equipment company and your home health or private duty company. Pricing varies, so I suggest you exercise your right to choose and not just accept any company you are referred to. It may not provide the best results for your needs, and may not be cost effective for you.

Private Residential Care Homes - The name pretty much describes this type of living and care arrangement. These are privately owned large homes that house and provide care for generally three to six residents.

Regulations vary by state, so more details are not included here. The feeling and care in private residential care homes is more like home and family. Average costs are between $1,500 and $4,500 per month but can be higher depending on the area and the care home. It's important to check out the qualifications and backgrounds of the owner and staff, and inquire how they handle medical problems and emergencies.

Assisted Living Facilities (ALFs) - These facilities differ in their offerings and living quarters. Rooms can range from studio apartments to full-sized apartments with kitchenettes. The cost varies with the type and size of the room. You choose your level of care from options such as two or more meals daily, care management and monitoring, help with activities of daily living (ADLs) such as showering, grooming, going to the bathroom, transferring to and from wheelchairs. Other services include housekeeping, laundry, medication management, recreational activities, transportation to group events , and possibly beauty shop services. Higher-end assisted living facilities offer massage, aromatherapy, and spa services. Security varies by facility also, but my experience is that most are providing at least some level of security. Care options are not included in the base price: there are varying *a la carte* charges for care services and assistance.

ALFs do not have physicians on staff and only provide basic medication management; none offer medical care. Residents are responsible for their own phones and transportation to doctor appointments and medical care outside of the facility. Some facilities may offer free cable TV or internet access. Regulations regarding ALFs vary by state. As an example, Michigan does not require a registered nurse on staff. Staff requirements and state licensing is different than for skilled nursing facilities.

Skilled Nursing Home - Skilled nursing homes are either private or a combination of private and public, meaning they designate beds for private pay patients and Medicaid patients. Private beds can be paid for by private insurance and often are, but cannot be utilized by patients on Medicaid. Other than the rehab portion mentioned above, Medicare does not pay for long-term skilled care. Skilled nursing care operates much the same as rehab care but with long-term care needs in mind. It is considered medical care and has much more stringent regulations and requirements than the ALFs or residential facilities do. Keep in mind that the facilities that had the serious neglect issues I mentioned were skilled nursing homes under the strictest state requirements, which tells you how much that means. They offer therapy and social work services, but not with an immediate goal of improving the patient to independence and discharge.

Some skilled nursing homes also may have a number of respite beds which hospice companies contract for their patients on a very short term basis. Families can usually utilize respite beds through hospice if they are full-time caregivers and need a break for a vacation or other short-term need. In 2011, MetLife reported the average cost of skilled nursing homes to be $78,110 to $87,235 a year for a semi-private room. Under Medicare, you would pay over $11,000 for days 21 to 100 and then be responsible for 100% of the rest of the year, or approximately $56,000 more, and that's provided Medicare covered you post hospitalization.

I don't spend $78,000 a year to live in my home now, let alone a ten-by-ten foot space with at least one other person! If we live to the current life expectancy of seventy-eight years, we would need over $1 million dollars for skilled nursing care in a shared room! Many of us will live well beyond seventy-eight. Just five years of care costs nearly $400,000. Are you preparing for that?

Home care -

Home Health Care - Home health care is intermittent medical care provided in the home for homebound patients. It is a benefit of Medicare, Medicaid, and most private health insurances if the patient meets specific criteria. Home health care provides nursing, physical therapy, occupational therapy, speech therapy, social work services, and home health aides.

Patients who qualify typically have had an acute health change requiring hospitalization, and home health care is initiated upon hospital discharge. The patient must be homebound, meaning they only leave their home with assistance for medical appointments or religious services. Recent hospitalization is not required, but that is the most common qualifier for home health care. A patient can also qualify if there is a significant change in health status, such as an acute illness or injury not requiring hospitalization. For example, if a patient went to a hospital emergency department for trouble breathing, and was having a hard time controlling congestive heart failure, he would most likely qualify for home health care, but he would have to be homebound. Patients who become physically debilitated due to an illness or injury and need therapy to regain strength and balance may also qualify. Patients can also qualify based on a new life-altering diagnosis, such as insulin-dependent diabetes. Diabetics are at risk for a multitude of problems from uncontrolled blood sugar, so education and monitoring is essential to prevent complications.

Home health care is always set up on a short-term, temporary basis for what is called a "60-day certification period." The physician must order nursing care or physical therapy to obtain home health care coverage by Medicare, Medicaid, or private insurance. The nurse typically determines which of the available services will be initiated and how often the nurse and the home health aide will visit. Therapists conduct their own evaluation to determine the frequency and length of their visits, unless the physician orders a specific number of visits per week.

The goal of home health care is to improve health outcomes. The services are guided by Medicare Guidelines. Medicare expects the home health care team to educate the patient and family about the patient's diagnosis and treatment and to discharge the patient as soon as possible. Medical procedures such as dressing changes on wounds, daily catheterization, and injections that were once done by nurses are now being taught to patients and families with the expectation that a responsible family member or friend will perform those procedures.

Home health aides can only provide personal care according to Medicare guidelines. This includes bathing and grooming, but does not include providing meals, housekeeping, or any type of task that isn't directly related to personal care.

Therapists provide therapy, but their main job is to educate the patient about what to do, and all the work is up to the patient. No patient really improves if they don't follow the therapist's directions and exercise plan when the therapist is not there.

There is always a care plan that is followed by the team, with the inclusion of the patient and family if applicable. The professionals who visit will typically be in the home for forty-five minutes to an hour per visit. As weeks progress in the 60-day certification period, the frequency of visits decreases unless the patient's health status declines. If the team determines the patient improves to the point where she no longer qualifies for services or does not remain homebound, the team will discharge the patient before the 60-day certification period ends. If the patient continues to have significant health needs that cannot be improved in the 60-day period, the home health care team can re-certify the patient beyond 60 days.

Private Duty Home Care - Private duty home care is nonmedical care. The services are provided by caregivers or certified home health aides, depending on state regulations. The services provided are considered custodial care and do not require a physician's order. Services are designed to help the patient remain in their home as independently as possible or to provide respite for family caregivers by providing assistance with hygiene, meals, light housekeeping, companionship, errands, and medication reminders. Some private duty agencies transport clients, some do not.

Services are determined by the patient and the family, because private duty care is not covered by health insurance. Most private duty homecare services are paid out of pocket, but they may be covered in part or whole by Long-Term Care Insurance or Veterans benefits. Individual states may have programs providing limited private duty home care for low-income residents, but in my experience, the number of residents who can qualify for services is very limited. There is typically a waiting list for these programs or they are closed to new applicants. The agencies that contract with them provide very limited services.

As a previous homecare agency owner, I never participated in the Medicaid Waiver Program, as it's called in Michigan. Because the reimbursement rate is so low, I would have had to personally cover a portion of the patients' care. Agencies that contract for these services typically pay their caregiver's a very low wage and therefore don't attract or retain the best staff. My agency paid a higher wage to attract and hire the best caregivers possible. Check with your local or state Department of Aging for programs available in your area. Funding cuts are being made on a regular basis, so they may be very different now than a year ago.

Private duty care often works in collaboration with home health agencies or hospice because the services are different. Typically, if someone needs home health, they also need assistance with activities of daily living (ADLs). Because I am a nurse and geriatric care manager, I always assessed the need for home health care if our clients came to us before a home health agency. I made referrals so that our clients could improve to the best quality of life possible. Many private duty agencies do not involve themselves with health care at all, because most private duty agencies are not owned or directed by health care professionals and thus lack the necessary knowledge and understanding of health care needs.

Private duty home care is available 24 hours a day/365 days a year. Clients can obtain services long-term or short-term. Some agencies require a minimum amount of hours per shift, per day, or per week. This varies by agency, as do the rates, so check around.

Each state determines whether to regulate private duty agencies, so check with your state to determine whether they license private duty agencies or not. My home state of Michigan is an unlicensed state. Ethical, legitimate agencies like mine have pushed for regulation for the protection of the elderly, and those issues are now being discussed in the House and Senate of many unlicensed states.

Private duty agencies may use independent contractors or hire employees to provide care, but they cannot offer both. This is part of the reason for the huge range of costs, in addition to the regional cost of living. If an agency provides an independent contractor, they are not responsible for providing workman's compensation, unemployment insurance, or deducting employee taxes. They have far less control than employee-structured agencies, but it comes with a cost.

Private duty agencies are not certified by Medicare, because Medicare does not cover these services. Agencies that have both home health and private duty may appear to be certified to provide private duty care, but they are not. This can be misleading to the general public and to those who work in healthcare but are unfamiliar with the differences.

Long-term care insurance companies have been difficult to deal with in recent years because their policies state that the home care agency must be licensed or Medicare certified. Insurance companies are beginning to understand that this certification varies by state, and Medicare doesn't certify nonmedical care, so they are beginning to pay claims they tried to deny in the past. My agency had battled a few long-term care insurance companies over paying for clients' benefits. If you carry long-term care insurance or are considering a policy, read every single word and do some investigating into the company's history and consumer-satisfaction rating. This is easily obtained by doing a Google search with the insurance company's name plus the word *complaints*.

Continuing Care Retirement Communities (CCRC) - CCRCs comprise a combination of independent, semi-independent, and skilled care. I refer to it as step-down care. CCRCs operate using a buy-in philosophy that helps individuals move to different levels of care as their needs change. These communities typically charge an entrance fee and then charge additionally according to the level of care required. Residents may move into an apartment or condo as a healthy independent person. As they age, or if they acquire serious health problems or sustain injuries, they are able to move to an assisted–living facility for access to more services and skilled nursing care. The theory is that an individual can move easily from one level to another but may have to wait for an available bed. CCRCs can be very expensive and are not for middle- and low-income individuals. Members of the community are given priority over the general public.

Very few companies that offer both home health and private duty care do both well. Focus tends to be on the home health division with little attention to providing excellent private duty. Some companies are becoming all-inclusive conglomerates that offer everything from independent-living condos to skilled nursing homes, plus rehab, home health, and private duty. But, again, they don't seem to do it all well, and they are more fragmented than they appear. I have known of companies in which the quality of care is so uneven that discharge planners in one area won't refer to other areas of the same company because the quality doesn't meet the expectations they have for their patients. But, believe me, they are pressured by the company to only refer within. Don't assume that if a company has a great home health care component, they also offer a great rehab or skilled nursing facility. I would rather contract a company whose concentration and expertise is in one area—such as private duty or home health—than a company that tries to do it all.

Hospice - Hospice provides end-of-life care for people who are dying and support services for their families. Hospice can be provided in homes, hospice facilities, long-term care facilities, and hospitals. Medicare, Medicaid, and most private health care insurance companies cover hospice care. Coverage for hospice care requires a physician's order based on a terminal diagnosis, but does not require the patient to be homebound. Previously, patients became eligible for hospice when they were expected to live six months or less. That is no longer the case. Although imminent death is a criteria, hospice care is provided when curative care is no longer possible or desired.

Hospice provides care from nurses, home health aides, social workers, spiritual care providers, volunteers who perform a variety of tasks, and bereavement counselors who may provide individual and group support for up to one year following the patient's death. Patients may use all or some of the services based on their needs and preferences. Visits are short, typically from forty-five minutes to one and a half hours. If the patient is in need of pain control or other comfort measures, nurses may be in the home longer. If other needs exist, volunteers may visit more frequently and stay for a longer period of time.

Although hospice operates under the supervision of a primary care physician or a medical director who is a physician, hospice nurses direct the care. Nurses work with other hospice professionals, family members, and sometimes the patient's friends using a team approach to provide palliative—or comfort—care.

Some home health care agencies also offer hospice services. They often have a transition, or bridge, program. Patients may start out with home health care, and as their health declines and a cure becomes unlikely or impossible, they may decide to transition to hospice services. Patients never receive both types of care at the same time. The focus of home health care and hospice are very different. Home health care concentrates on improvement while hospice concentrates on palliative, or comfort, care. Hospice specializes in pain control and the process of dying. It addresses the physical, emotional, and spiritual needs of the patient and also the family and close friends.

Private duty care often works in collaboration with hospice to provide care when families are unable to or need respite. Private duty care follows the direction of the hospice team to maintain comfort and support for the patient. Rather than contacting emergency services or the patient's physician for direction when changes in the patient's health status occur, private-duty caregivers contact the hospice nurse for instructions.

The vast majority of seniors want to remain in their homes. Do you want to live in a nursing home? What are you going to do to prevent that? We must break the old-school thought patterns of how we view aging and what we expect for our elderly family members and ourselves. There are doable models of housing and services that can respond to crises, reduce costs, and improve care. I will describe such a model in Part 3.

Socialization

It is important to discuss the socialization of the aging population because there has been a drastic change in the last thirty to forty years. It wasn't that many years ago when families remained in close proximity and neighbors were friendly and helpful. The aging population was cared for in large part by their loved ones. In some parts of the world, this remains true. But not in the U.S.

In an essay titled "The Transformation of American Family Structure," published in *American Historical Review* in 1994, Steven Ruggles wrote that in 1880, approximately seventy-five percent of U.S. Caucasians age sixty-five and older lived with a family member. By 1980, that figure dropped to less than twenty-five percent.

We now live in a society where the vast majority of women work, our life expectancy is increasing, and relocating for a job or other reasons is commonplace. Neighbors may be too busy working, raising children, and trying to do it all to check in or provide assistance on a frequent basis. That leaves the sixty-five-and-older crowd on their own to meet their socialization needs.

People who live in senior communities have more opportunities for making friends, participating in activities, and socializing over meals. Those who remain in their homes as married or partnered couples may not have many friends. What can they do to socialize if they are alone or their spouse dies? If they lead an active life, are healthy, and can still drive, it will be easier to maintain friendships and participate in social activities. But many elderly people sit alone, day after day, without seeing or talking to another human being. It seems likely that people who remain in their homes alone will easily fall into a lonely existence, but it happens in long-term care facilities, too. Whether due to shyness, lack of interest, or depression, there are seniors living very lonely existences surrounded by people.

As I've mentioned previously, we don't change the core of who we are as our birthdays pass. If you were shy or outgoing when you were younger, you will likely be that way in your senior years, unless you are affected by depression, dementia, or another brain disease. Some people go through life having one or two close friends, others have many friends, and some are just loners. If you lose the one or two close friends you have, can you imagine trying to replace those friendships when you are in your seventies or eighties? It is far more difficult to make friends when you are out of the work force and live alone in your home. The need for social interaction and a feeling of belonging and worth are still important, just less easily obtained.

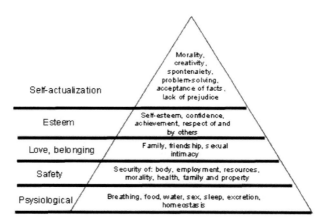

If you've ever taken a psychology class, you most likely encountered Abraham Maslow's "Hierarchy of Needs." Maslow believed that our motivations are based on five levels of needs which are typically displayed in a pyramid, the most basic needs at the bottom. According to Maslow's theory, the needs of each lower level must be satisfied before a person may begin striving to fulfill the needs of the next higher level. For example, people must meet their basic needs for air, food, water, and shelter before striving for security of employment, health, and property. Only when that level's needs are secured will people pursue family, friendships, and sexual intimacy, and so on up the pyramid.

Can you see the importance of socialization and feeling secure? What happens to us when we lose those important aspects of our lives? Imagine you are in your eighties with failing health and no friends or family because they have died or live too far away to visit or assist you. Imagine not being hugged or touched for months or even years. Can you? Many elderly people live with no socialization or physical contact with other people whatsoever.

Even seniors living in nursing homes, surrounded by people, can long to hear a kind word or wish for someone to acknowledge them as worthy. The Geriatric Mental Health Foundation (GMHF) fact sheet on depression reports that fifteen out of every one hundred persons age sixty-five or older is depressed. That's six million out of the forty million people age sixty-five and older. Even more staggering is the estimate by the GMHF that upwards of fifty percent of nursing-home residents are depressed. The lowest rates of depression in seniors are among those living in communities.

Much of society views depression as some sadness, but it is much more than that. An entire book could be devoted to just this topic and the difference between situational depression and clinical depression, but a summarized list of symptoms of clinical depression below shows that depression is more than just a case of sadness.

Most are surprised that the highest rates of suicide are among those sixty-five and older compared with any other age group. The National Institutes of Health online publication titled "Older Adults: Depression and Suicide Facts" (NIH Publication No. 4593, last revised April 2007) states: "14.3 of every 100,000 people age 65 and older died by suicide in 2004, higher than the rate of about 11 per 100,000 in the general population."

Depression is not a normal part of aging. Depression in the elderly is also under-recognized and under-treated. Depression should always be considered if one or more of the following are displayed:

Persistent sadness lasting two or more weeks

Difficulty sleeping or concentrating

Feeling slowed down

Withdrawal from regular social activities

Excessive worry about finances and health problems

Pacing and fidgeting

Feeling worthless or helpless

Changes in weight or appearance

Frequent tearfulness

Thoughts of suicide or death

Depression is treatable, and successful treatment can make a world of difference in an elderly person's quality of life. However, we need to consider prevention. If seniors who live in nursing homes are more depressed than those who live in their community, then we must consider feasible alternatives, which I discuss in Part 3 of this book.

If you are reading this book and you are a family member or professional caregiver of an elderly person, think about your role in brightening the day of the person you care for. Think about Maslow's hierarchy of needs and what you can do to make your loved one or your patient feel loved, secure, worthy, and engaged. A kind word, a smile, a hug, and a willingness to listen can do wonders for their mental and physical health. Try to leave them happier than you found them. These simple gestures will improve your health and outlook as well. Meeting the needs of others, according to Maslow's theory, will meet our own needs for love and esteem. Treating others as you would like to be treated is a win-win situation! I can't begin to tell you how rewarded I feel by the work I do. Overhearing a patient or family member remark, "She is so nice," or "She is a great nurse," is more satisfying than almost anything I can think of. It's not because I want to hear how great I am, but because those words tell me I left them better than I found them. I did something to improve their day. Don't we all want to feel needed and valued?

Throughout the book I am offering different perspectives for you to consider. Bringing you to an empathetic point of view is one of my primary intentions of this book and my work. Empathy can be better understood by introducing different thoughts and perspectives which may have not been considered before. If you are a care provider have you thought about the birth of your loved one or the births of your elderly patients? I cared for patients for nearly 30 years before I thought about the births of my patients, and it was like a light bulb moment in a hospital room following the birth of one of my grandchildren. The perspective impacted me so much, and took so long to come into my own care perceptions that I'd like to share it.

Not only is it important to think about the history of the care recipient, but I think it's also important to think about them from their mother's perspective. If you are a care provider, the person you care for has or had a mother. That mother undoubtedly loved her child like no other. If you've ever had a child, you know the tremendous love you felt when your baby arrived. Your care recipient's mother also had hopes and dreams for her baby's future.

As a mother of two adult sons, three adult stepchildren, and four grandchildren, I know what I hope for all of them: nothing but great things. That hope will never stop. Whether I am here or not, I want the best for all of them, throughout their entire lives. So as you care for an elder, remember that their mother also wanted the best for them. Take a moment to think about her love for her now elderly child. Be the person that you would want to take care of your child, young or old. Acknowledge the person's life prior to their loss of memory and independence. Understand that they deserve nothing less than the best you have to give. It is an enormous honor to care for someone. You have been trusted with their care. When providing care, ask yourself how you would want your child cared for, and let that guide the care you provide. Give your care recipient the best. The best care always comes from a place of empathy. Not only do I recommend putting yourself in the shoes of the persons you care for, but add to that by putting yourself in their mothers' shoes, too.

As cliché as it is, we receive what we give. I promise that if you always try to put yourself in the shoes of the person you care for, you will always provide the best care you can and will feel good about what you are doing.

The state of Medicare, Medicaid, Social Security, and other programs

I made some references to current concerns about Medicare and Social Security in earlier chapters. Let's look now at the frightening reality of it all.

The numbers are out. The articles and endless news reports are everywhere. We cannot afford to support the eighty million citizens who will be sixty-five and older by the year 2030. Medicare won't keep up with the rapidly increasing health-care costs and our expanding life expectancy. A 2010 New York Times article titled "Social Security to See Payout Exceed Pay-In This Year" stated that the "system will pay out more in benefits than it receives in payroll taxes, an important threshold it was not expected to cross until at least 2016, according to the Congressional Budget Office." The Social Security Bulletin (vol. 66, No. 4; p. 37) states the ratio of workers paying into Social Security for every one person drawing out was 5.1 in 1960, 3.3 in 2005, and will be down to 2.6 by 2020. The article stated, "With currently scheduled tax rates and benefits, the system needs a worker-to-beneficiary ratio of about 2.8 to function at a pay-as-you-go level (meaning that tax revenue approximately equals benefit payments)." We are currently in the midst of a negative ratio as 2020 is drawing near.

Disappearing pension plans, diminishing personal savings, hefty losses in the stock market, and loss of home equity in recent years have all contributed to more Americans relying on Social Security alone for their retirement. Drawn from a survey on CareerBuilder.com in 2009, thirty-six percent of Americans don't contribute anything at all to a retirement plan, according to the follow-up article by CNBC titled "More Upper-Income Workers Living Paycheck to Paycheck."

According to Representative Fred Upton in his blog posted on The Hill, "The Medicare trust fund will run dry in 2024, five years earlier than last year's estimate." In 2010, Medicare expenditures reached $523 billion, but the income was only $486 billion, leaving a $37 billion deficit in just one year.

Costs are rising, and the funding for retirement programs we paid into are on the brink of collapse. Our legislators can't agree on solutions. We are facing the biggest population of retirees our nation has ever seen. So, what does this mean for us all? What the heck are we going to do? It's a disaster in progress!

Americans are forgoing preventative medicine or delaying treatment for lack of insurance or the ability to pay huge deductibles and co-pays. People are upside down in their mortgages or losing their homes to foreclosure. Many employees feel insecure in their jobs as corruption in business grows. Small businesses are being lost to increasing taxes and insurance costs. Industries that were big, stable, and successful in the past are now struggling, downsizing, or closing altogether.

I know I am not the only one who feels that almost nothing now is secure and can be counted on. The retirement funds I planned on outside of Medicare and Social Security have been hugely affected by the economic downturn. What I counted on simply isn't there. I bet it's a rare individual who reads this book and feels totally secure about their financial future as they think of their retirement years. How do you feel, right now, about your ability to support and care for yourself in your sixties, seventies, and eighties? Ten years ago, I was sure I'd be okay, but unless I act now to secure another plan, and you act too, we will not be okay.

There is hope in the midst of what seems hopeless if we expand our thinking and decide to act now! In Part 3, I will describe a new way of living and caring for the elderly. But now, I am going to introduce you to people who are living the current reality.

Part 2   *Behind the Old Face*

Chapter 5
What is *Behind the Old Face?*

I described in Part 1 how and when the title came to me, but not the importance of *Behind the Old Face* and what it means to the purpose of this book, to the greater project, and to you as a reader. *Behind the Old Face* is self-evident as far as I'm concerned, but it may not be as evident to those outside of the world of eldercare or to those who are new to it.

I am saddened as I think about the times I have heard a senior say, "I feel like a number," or, "I feel as if I don't matter; I'm just old and tossed aside." Where does that come from? What is the perception of younger adults when they see the outward appearance of the lines of time on a face? We all have an opinion on using the word *old* in the description of aging. I have heard people in their eighties, including my late grandma, describe other residents where they live as "those old people." The title *Behind the Old Face* is in no way meant to be disrespectful. I have said "I love old people" hundreds if not thousands of time with the most genuine regard and respect. The title describes the life beyond what you see when you look into the face of an aging adult, because there is so much more to a person than their facial appearance. The perception of what an old face represents is what needs to change. An old face shouldn't be perceived as useless, something to discard, or past its time of value. How many of us love our old pair of jeans or those old worn out comfortable shoes? We see value in those, and they can't compare to the true value of an elderly person, so we just need to understand there is more *Behind the Old Face* that is of much value to us all.

The lives behind the old faces

Part 2 includes real stories and situations from people I have met, cared for, and interviewed specifically for this book. The people you will meet and get to know in the following pages were not specifically chosen based on their background or story; it was only through interviews that I learned about them and their lives. Some I met through their contact with my homecare agency, others were living in local facilities and agreed to be a part of this book. Others whom I have cared for or have somehow been in their lives even for a brief time are described with a fictitious name to protect their privacy.

Even though I have spent over thirty years involved in the lives of the elderly, I found myself surprised and amazed by some of the stories I heard and who these people were. As you read on, think about the fact that these people are our neighbors. They live in our neighborhoods, in local senior care facilities, and they stand next to us in the grocery store line or sit beside us in the waiting room of a doctor's office. Do you really know who you are looking at when you see an old face or meet an aging adult?

Those whom I interviewed gave me permission to use their photos, names, and the information about their lives, thoughts, opinions, and situations. It has been a privilege and an honor to have met them, spent time with them, and been allowed into some of their deepest thoughts, feelings, and lives so that we can all understand there is more *Behind the Old Face*. You will see a facial image of many of the people I interviewed for this book. Take a moment to really look at their faces prior to reading about their lives. Ask yourself what your thoughts and feelings are when their faces are all you see, and then ask yourself again after you read their stories.

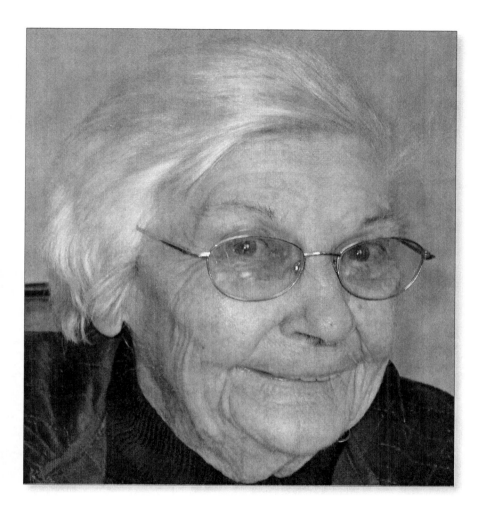

Marian Grace - To be alone or not to be alone?

Early in 2011, I met Marian after receiving a phone call from her nephew, who lived out of state, about providing some homecare services for his aunt. He went on to say that Marian no longer drove and her only family lived out of state. We carried on the conversation before he told me Marian wasn't too receptive about receiving help and had just thrown out the last couple of people who tried to help her. Since he and his wife were the only involved family, and they lived so far away, he had concerns for her well-being. This is a very typical phone call from a loving, concerned family member. No one wants to lose independence and accept help. Who can blame them? On the other hand, it's very worrisome for families who can't visit frequently to assist or make sure their aging loved one is okay and safe.

I had concerns whether Marian would accept help after what her nephew revealed, but I have a particular soft spot for the tough ones, so I called Marian. She was not what I expected. We had a very pleasant telephone conversation and she agreed to meet. I took an instant liking to Marian, and we had a wonderful visit! I kept what her nephew said in the back of my mind, but couldn't imagine her throwing anyone out. After a bit of prodding, Marian allowed me to help her with a grocery list and to add some much needed nutritional items, and I went shopping following our visit. Typically, I would speak with my office staff and we would schedule a caregiver to assist, but since she was in need of food and we hit it off, I decided to take care of it myself. This is the difference between a company that truly cares about helping people and those whose main focus is financial gain. How many company owners would grocery shop or personally visit and assist an elderly client?

I had some concerns about Marian being alone, so I discussed a personal emergency response system with her and her family, and she approved the purchase and installation. This eased her family's mind and mine. I found myself thinking about Marian a lot. I thought about her being alone all the time except for her family visits every few weeks and my visits, since I decided to provide her grocery shopping myself. Marian was sweet and so grateful for my calls, visits, and assistance that I had a hard time understanding why she had dismissed others who attempted to help her.

Marian readily agreed to being interviewed for this book, although she couldn't understand for the life of her why I would be interested in her story. Marian was one of the few people I videotaped during the interviews, because the initial intent of the interviews and stories were only for this book. I began working with Jared Rosen, the founder of DreamSculpt, and decided to create an M2ebook™ prior to the publication of this book. Marian's interview had not yet taken place, and video clips were necessary for the M2ebook™ titled, *The Aging Question: A Vision for the Coming Elder Boom*. Although the video clips of Marian are short, I have a video of the entire interview that I love to watch. I wish I had video recorded all of the interviews, because they warm my heart when I see them.

Marian is a strong and independent woman. She celebrated her eighty-eighth birthday on New Year's Eve 2011. Marian is one of the few seniors I've met without any medical problems. She smokes like crazy and likes a beer now and then. She has a deep voice and a great sense of humor. In many way, I see myself in Marian. I will do it myself, get along without help, and be just fine. Marian always said to me, "I am just fine." Marian seemed to have more concern about how much I worked and the amount of rest I got than she did with her own lack of socialization, inability to get out of the house without help, or how she could tend to an urgent need.

I learned during the interview that Marian wasn't opposed to help, even though she didn't think she needed it. She threw the others before me out because they brought their problems and drama to her and wore her out with their complaints. Marian and I got along well because, as she said, "You really listen to me and care." I wonder how many people perceive seniors as difficult, uncooperative, and even aggressive without any consideration for their own approach, attitude, and behavior. This is not uncommon. Thousands of seniors have been drugged for behavior problems in nursing homes, sent in for psychiatric evaluations, and been calmed down by psychiatric medications at home because of pushy and disrespectful care providers. Being stripped of dignity and independence, or hurried into actions that you don't want to do or when you are not ready, would cause you to react in anger, yet the behavior is blamed on the care recipient rather than the care provider's demeanour and approach.

It makes me think about *Super Nanny* coming to the rescue of parents with unruly children when it really is about the parents' inability to recognize the needs of their children and to appropriately interact and talk with their kids. I want to be the *Super Friend of Seniors* and teach care providers how to better approach, talk to, and care for aging adults without drugging them and making their lives miserable!

As I continue with Marian's story, and more stories of aging adults, see if you can recognize their needs. Can you see how much better their lives could be if those needs were met? Put yourself in their shoes. How would you feel in similar situations and circumstances? What would you want from the people in your life or from professional care providers? If you were alone most of the time, and the regular visits you received were from negative complainers, how long would you want them to stay? Personally, I am not alone and I have declared my home a drama-free zone. We all have enough to deal with without having constant complainers in our lives. Can you now see why Marian threw them out? Do you see why I couldn't imagine that happening? It wasn't Marian. She didn't have the problem! Marian just reacted to the intrusion of peace and comfort in her life.

Marian grew up in Ypsilanti, Michigan, and lived there her whole life until September 2011 when she moved out of state to live with her nephew and his wife. Marian was raised in a large family of seven brothers and sisters. Her dad died when she was eleven years old. She wanted to be a nurse when she was young, but the family couldn't afford college. Her older brother and sister helped Marian go to cosmetology school, but Marian didn't remain in that profession because the income wasn't stable. She said, "I could be at work all day but not get my first client until 4:00 or 5:00 in the afternoon, so it just wasn't secure."

Throughout the interview, Marian's eyes sparkled when she talked of her mom and how strong her mother was through the colon cancer which ended her life. The eyes are very telling, because through them you can see the recollection of memories, love, joy, humor, sadness, and pain.

Even though Marian never became a professional nurse, she and her sisters cared for their mother through her illness. Marian also cared for her husband through lung cancer before he passed away. Nursing is about caring for other human beings, so even though Marian didn't get the educational background and degree she wanted, her contribution to others fulfilled her desire to help people. The word *nursing* is derived from the thirteenth-century Latin word *nutrire*, which means "to nourish." The current meaning evolved over the years, but I think the sixteenth-century definition is more at the core of what a nurse is—nurse: "a person, usually a woman, who waits upon or tends to the sick." In that sense, Marian was a nurse.

Marian lost the two most important men in her life at young ages. She was fifty-two years old when she lost her husband of twenty-five years. Loss at any age is difficult, but losing a father at the young age of eleven and a husband before retirement age is never expected. In many ways, Marian has the strength she admired in her mother without realizing that she is as admirable.

Marian worked for a printing company for twenty-five years before retiring at age sixty-two. The company changed in a way she felt was not good and far from how it was when she started. She retired with the perspective of looking back rather than forward, saying, "It was more about leaving a job I no longer liked than looking forward to the years ahead." Marian told me the best thing about retirement is being able to do as you please.

Marian remained healthy and independent but said, "Losing the ability to get around like I used to is what's difficult." She only recently recognized her decrease in mobility, and that is when she really started to "feel" old.

Most of the questions I posed to Marian about aging were very comfortable for her to answer. She said she occasionally thinks about how long she can remain in her home or she will live, but she has no fear. The interview took place just a couple months prior to her move to North Carolina to live with her nephew and his wife. At that time, the move was planned for the winter months only.

When I asked Marian about how she thinks the elderly are treated, she said, "Old people are neglected. They are treated by the majority of people like just a number. The majority of people just don't care about old people." She went on to say, "If people cared as much as you do, old people would live out their lives very good at the end." Isn't it sad that from Marian's perspective and that of many others I've talked with, few people care about the elderly? We're always talking about discrimination as if it is only experienced because of race, sexual orientation, gender, or religion, but seniors experience discrimination on a regular and widespread basis.

I asked Marian what she thinks we could do as a society to improve the treatment and care of the elderly, and she said, "It starts with kids. Kids need to be raised respecting old people." She then began to elaborate on how much she liked me because, "You are a listener. You didn't just barge in and plop down and talk about yourself and your problems. You really listened to me." Marian believes this is an important factor in the unsatisfactory treatment and care of the elderly, and I have to agree with her. It all comes back to feeling valued. I have seen care providers talk with the family over seniors about their health or care, as if they weren't even there, even though the senior was fully alert and capable of talking, understanding, answering questions, and making their own decisions.

If you think about yourself, how do you feel when your thoughts, feelings, opinions, and communications are ignored or unheard? Do you think that changes as you age? If anything, we need to be more attentive to the aging population when we have the opportunity, because they do lack the social-ization and opportunities to be heard on a regular basis. Imagine Marian liv-ing alone for the last twenty-eight years as a retiree. Imagine losing friends and contact with friends as the years go by. That is an incredible amount of time to be alone to think with little opportunity to be heard. Marian cut off or significantly reduced contact with friends in the past prior to my meeting her because they brought nothing but complaints, negativity, and problems to her. She said she'd rather be alone than be worn out by listening for hours to someone else's problems. Can you blame her? Marian does not lack concern or care for others. She regularly voiced concern about the time and effort her niece and nephew put into caring for her and about my workload. The dif-ference is that we bring something positive to the relationship, because our focus is not on ourselves, it is on her. This is important to recognize in all our relationships, but it is exceptionally important when coming in contact with or caring for aging adults who have fewer and fewer relationships as they age.

Many seniors have so little contact and socialization, you may be the only person they see or talk to for days, weeks, or even months. Whether con-tact means a one-time conversation over the phone for business, occa-sional face-to-face contact in a doctor's office or pharmacy, a professional caregiving relationship, or a distant or close family relationship, it's im-portant to take note of what we bring to those in need of kindness, care, respect, socialization, and feeling valued.

Dr. Phil always says, "You either contribute to or contaminate a relation-ship." Relationships come in all sizes and forms, and we only have to think about how we feel on the receiving end of someone's words and attitude to understand how we should approach and treat an elderly person. It seems so simple to just treat people the way you'd like to be treated, but it is a rare person who always treats every single person who crosses their path as they'd liked to be treated. This seems less so with the elderly, because we have a harder time relating and seeing their perspective. Empathy isn't a skill that can be taught, but I do believe we can evoke empathy or increase our empathy by getting to know people, their life history, and their point of view. Even when a senior has aphasia and can't talk, or dementia and can't remember or respond appropriately, we need to know more about their lives and how to best communicate with them in a respectful, dignified manner. People with aphasia have difficulty with language, not intelligence, yet care providers often treat them as if they don't comprehend, when nothing could be further from the truth.

Since Marian moved to her niece and nephew's home in North Carolina, I occasionally get e-mails from her niece with updates and photos of Marian. Marian appears to have a new and refreshed look of life and happiness. She is getting out in the world, socializing, and once again enjoying life. I cannot explain how wonderful it is to see the complete joy on her face. It is amazing and makes my heart truly happy. I suspect that Marian will not return to live alone in her little home in Ypsilanti, Michigan, and I hope she doesn't. Her niece and nephew have given her a true gift of happiness, love, inclusion, and value that has turned her very quiet, lonely years of sitting day after day alone in her little house to the good years she described in our interview. Life is about quality not quantity, as cliché as that may seem. Who wouldn't rather live sixty-five years happy than an additional twenty years miserable?

Marian is fortunate to have extended family who truly love her and opened their lives and home to her. Not everyone has a nephew and niece like Marian's. Not everyone has family or friends who provide assistance or care. On the other hand, not every senior living alone is willing to move to a safer and more social environment, even when there are concerned family and friends. I will tell you more stories in this part of the book that gave me great concern for the elderly people out there alone and unsafe. I'll finish Marian's story by telling you that her intention is to leave this world peacefully, because she's wanted only to be kind and never hurt anyone. That may seem like a rather simple goal and expectation compared with others who want to leave a huge mark on society, but Marian's expectation of herself and her life could not be more important.

As you stand in a grocery store line, or are slowed down by an elderly person in front of, you think about Marian. Wonder if the old face you are looking at has gone through such painful loss at an early age. Think about the career dreams they had when they were children. Think about how they may be living a life with the simple intention of just being kind, because you could be standing next to Marian.

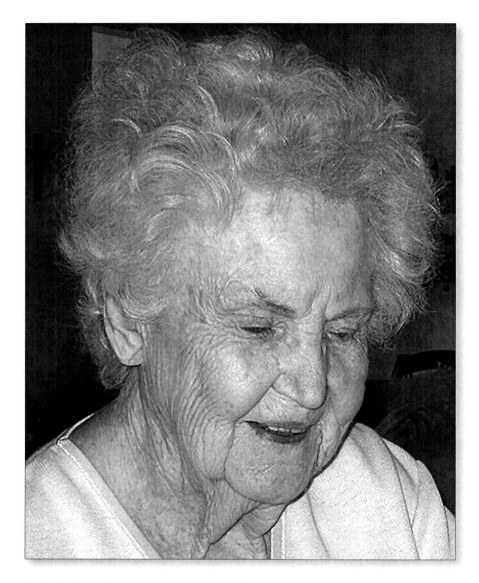

Left behind - Margaret Juzwiak's Story

Margaret, born June 9, 1922, is a very pleasant, good natured, and inter-esting lady. I have known Margaret since she called our agency for assis-tance in 2008. I got to know much more about her through inviting her to our home one Christmas and through interviewing her for this book, which I did by the way, on her eighty-ninth birthday in 2011. I started the interview by asking Margaret what she thought of aging. Her response was, "I hate it of course." She went on to say, "It's difficult to get around anymore. The aches and pains and arthritis are difficult when the weather isn't good." She talked about reducing her garden and the amount of flowers she had because it was too difficult to care for them any longer.

We chatted a bit about her flowers and her love of gardening, and then I asked Margaret what her aspirations were when she was a young girl. She said she wanted to go to art school. But school was too expensive, and her dad wanted her to keep art as a hobby and do something else to make a living. "He didn't really believe in educating the girls anyway. He thought the boys needed to be educated, but not the girls." Margaret said she got a scholarship for nursing school when she was a senior in high school, so that's why she went on to become a nurse. Margaret primarily worked as a pediatric nurse with tuberculosis patients during the time when personal protection such as HEPA masks didn't exist. She literally put her own life on the line to provide care to patients who were shunned from society like lepers.

Margaret and her husband, Bernie, lived a comfortable life raising their family in a nice four-bedroom home. That home was where she eventually cared for her mother. After her mother and mother-in-law passed away, her husband was gone, and her adult children were raising their own families, she sold her home and moved into the apartment I interviewed her in. She said the upkeep on her house got to be too much, and she had a hard time finding a trustworthy handyman that wouldn't take advantage of her, stating, "They usually take advantage of a woman living alone." She accepted the move and downsizing without a problem.

I brought up the fact that Margaret lived her life active and caring for everyone else as a nurse and mother and asked what it felt like going into retirement. She smiled and said, "I loved being a grandma, and now I'm a great-grandma." She suddenly stopped and took a long pause, losing the smile she just had on her face. I could see the thoughts racing in her mind as I looked into her eyes. Then sadness blanketed her face as she said, "Things just went downhill after I lost my husband." Margaret's husband, Bernie, died suddenly at fifty-six of a heart attack at home after returning from a late meeting. Margaret was the same age as Bernie.

Bernie was a stock broker. Margaret said he took care of everything, referring to their finances, and when he died she knew very little about their financial picture and investments. She said that when her husband was away from work, he didn't want to talk about work because he spent so much time on the phone and paying attention to news and finances. "He just wanted to get away from it, and I couldn't blame him for that," she said.

Margaret was retired when she lost her husband. She retired in her late forties because her husband wanted her to travel with him. He traveled a lot for business and often won trips from meeting sales goals. Their kids were either already in college or near entering college at that time. As Margaret talked about her husband, it was very clear she had lost her best friend.

I asked Margaret what she missed most about being young. Her eyes lit up with a sparkle and she said, "I was always pretty active. I miss playing tennis, roller skating, ice skating, dancing . . . things like that. I especially miss swimming." Margaret gets around with a walker now. She stated she was falling a lot, and the cane just didn't help. I asked Margaret if she had a tough time adjusting to a walker. She said it didn't bother her because she focused on how to continue to get around rather than her loss and decline in mobility.

Many changes come with loss of mobility, but as mentioned in Part 1, it is our perspective that determines how well or poorly we adjust. Even though Margaret started off saying she hated aging because she can't get around like she used to, and throughout the interview it was very apparent that loss of mobility limits her and her independence, she accepts it as the natural progression of aging and continues to do what she is able within her limitations. Margaret hired assistance and is focusing on the satisfaction of remaining in her own home.

Margaret never let go of her dream to be an artist. Although she never made a career of it, she did paint and sold some of her pieces in craft shows when she was in her seventies and eighties. She drew live sketches at these events for a very small fee, which gave her just what she wanted: "the funds to buy more paint," she said with a giggle.

Margaret's apartment proudly displays her paintings. The small photo of her painting of a lighthouse is shown here in black and white for book-printing purposes. It doesn't do the justice its original color version deserves, but it does offer a 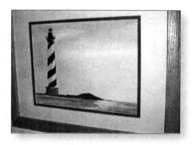 glimpse of Margaret's talent. Margaret honored me at the end of our day together by giving me a beautiful floral painting she created, which will be a treasure of mine for years to come.

Asking seniors I've interviewed for advice they want to pass on to those of us approaching our elder years is like getting a look from ahead on the mountain as we continue our trek towards that same place. Margaret didn't hesitate and said, "Everyone is so concerned about looking young and all this plastic surgery. There are so many things nowadays to take care of your skin and wrinkles by yourself, and you should just go along with the aging process because it's just a natural thing. Once you go against the natural laws of things, you are going to run into trouble." When I asked Margaret about her thoughts when she first saw her own grey hair and wrinkles, she chuckled and said, "Well, I started dying my hair early because my husband didn't have any grey hair, and I didn't want him looking younger than I did." She said, "Once my husband died, I didn't care anymore, I just let it go." She credits her mother's and mother-in-law's examples for her attitude toward aging. She said, "They never complained. They just took life as it came, worked as hard as they could, and did everything as long as they could."

Margaret and Bernie had a group of couples friends for over thirty years that they frequently went to dinner with. After her husband passed away, she didn't want to go to those dinners alone. She met a couple of gentlemen who would take her out to dinner just as friends. She met a divorced man who had wanted to go to seminary when he was younger. His plans were interrupted when his dad died, because he had to take over their farm. He went on to get married and have a family, but things weren't good so they divorced. She giggled as she said, "I felt safe with him since he wanted to go to seminary and I knew he didn't want to marry, and of course I wasn't going to get married again." They were very good friends. He moved one day to where his granddaughter lived, several hours away, and she never saw or heard from him again. She said that was okay.

Our conversation continued in a different direction about Margaret's thoughts regarding the soul and whether it ages. Margaret said, "I think the soul is life itself." She told me an old Irish saying she likes: "When a person dies, open the window so the soul can escape." Margaret seemed delighted by the thought. Her wonderful smile and the twinkle in her eyes had returned. She said, "That's the part of us that goes to heaven. One time, a nun told me we would see our family and friends when we go to heaven because that was our whole life on earth. That's something to look forward to." I had the distinct impression thoughts of Bernie were still deep in her mind. Margaret then shocked me with, "I tell friends I don't want to go to heaven, because then I'll have to see Bernie, and I don't know if I want to see him again." For that brief second I wondered if she was kidding, until she broke out in laughter and said, "I just say that to be funny."

Margaret said Bernie didn't have a sense of humor until he married her. "Then he had to, because of the silly stuff I pulled on him. He started to think it was funny and started pulling funny things on the people he worked with. He gained an Irish perspective, which made him get along with people better." I believe their humor gave them a very happy and joyous marriage, and they loved their time together because of it.

When I asked Margaret about her thoughts on the way seniors are treated, Margaret responded similarly to Marian saying, "I think they're neglected by family and friends, because they're not understood and no one knows what to do for them or how to care for them." It's interesting that Margaret responded in the third person rather than saying "we" are not understood. Margaret said, "It's great if you can stay in your own home with help, like I do. It's hard to depend on your family because they don't know what to do for you either." When I asked her what we could do to better understand how to care for seniors, she said, "It's difficult now because everyone has to work just to survive."

Margaret lives in an apartment that is not specifically for senior living. I asked her if she visits with neighbors or has friends nearby. She said she used to have a group of lady friends in her complex who got together once a month for breakfast. They started moving, one after the other, to higher-priced assisted living. Margaret looked into assisted living, but said it was all too expensive for her income, and she just couldn't afford it. She said she doesn't have enough in her savings, and she needs it available for an emergency. She went on to say, "I think I've just been too generous with my kids," as she rolled her eyes and smirked. Margaret now sees that she should have concerned herself with her own future rather than give her adult children money for cars and other things. A good lesson for the rest of us.

Her monthly rent is $1,200 for a two-bedroom apartment with no senior benefits or considerations. She said that is cheap for the area. Margaret said with a scoffed look, "The only thing I'd get with assisted living would be one meal a day and someone to do my laundry and clean my apartment. And it's over $2,000 a month. I can't live in a closet with a light for over $2,000 a month. I like living here on my own." Margaret said she can get her utilities and everything cheaper on her own, and she pays for the services from my agency with her long-term care insurance. She did say however, that she would have never bought the policy had she realized she would still have to pay the premiums of $4,000 a year even when she began to use the benefits. Note Margaret's lesson when considering retirement planning. Carefully read and understand the specifics of the policy if you plan on purchasing long-term care insurance.

Margaret is fortunate because she has Veterans Administration benefits that provide some monthly income and healthcare if she needs it. Currently, the VA and long-term care insurance policies are the only sources that will pay for nonmedical home care, which is what enables Margaret to remain independent in her home. We assist her with transportation to appointments, grocery shopping, errands, and some light housekeeping. She requires very little assistance to remain independent at home. We assist Margaret six hours a week. If Margaret did not have insurance or the ability to pay privately for assistance, she would have to rely on family and friends or be forced into a move that she does not want, such as a nursing home paid by Medicaid.

If we take the current average cost for nursing home care that Medicaid would pay for and subtract what it costs to assist Margaret six hours a week to remain at home, the government saves over $80,000 a year. Medicaid will not pay the $6,200 that enables seniors like Margaret to remain independent at home, but it will pay over $87,000 for 24-hour nursing home care. For the life of me, I cannot understand their rationale! Seniors typically do much better at home and stay healthier because they are not exposed to communicable diseases. They suffer less from depression or other causes of decline that so often happen to seniors living in nursing homes. What sense does that make? No wonder Medicare and Medicaid are going broke!

We continued our discussion about how Margaret spends her days and her thoughts about the future. She watches locals walking their dogs and children running to the apartment complex swimming pool through her window. I think there is a special simplicity in that, which typically isn't appreciated when we are young. Do you think that the children running by in their swimsuits remind Margaret of her younger days and her love of swimming? Is it her life on rewind? Can you see how those children resemble who Margaret was at one time and how they will one day become Margaret, looking into their own pasts? In many ways, we begin our lives with such simplicity and we end them in the same way.

Have you ever thought about when or if you will lose the ability to dream? I can tell you after spending time with thousands of seniors that dreams and desires don't go away. They may not be something that can be attained for one reason or another, but they don't go away. It makes me wonder if dreams are somehow attached to our souls. I asked Margaret if there was something she still wanted to do or accomplish, and she told me her sister wants to take her on a cruise to the Bahamas. The only thing stopping her from going is the difficulty with her mobility. She talked fondly of taking her thirteen-year-old granddaughter on a cruise many years ago and "what a ball" they had. Another cruise with her sister was also in her fond-memories bank. Margaret's sister is younger, and they don't see each other much, since her sister lives in New Mexico. Travel is too much for Margaret anymore, which tells me we need to do a much better job of helping our elderly travel so they are able to visit with those they love in their last years.

The actual interview ended with my expressing my appreciation for all Margaret shared and a suggestion to have some of the birthday cake I brought her. I am not sure who was more appreciative, me or Margaret. As she told me how happy she was that I came to spend the time with her, a tear fell from her eye. I'm not sure what affected Margaret most. Was it the small birthday acknowledgement, interest in her and her life, or the time she could bask in memories of love and joy? Whatever it was, I felt blessed by our time together. We had some birthday cake, and Margaret showed me around her apartment, pointing out the artwork she had painted. I left Margaret that day feeling such joy for knowing more about her and the privilege of being a part of her eighty-nine years.

Our society and the younger generations have become so self-absorbed. What I think we fail to recognize is that real happiness comes from giving, not taking. Giving a couple hours to Margaret that day was so much more joyful than anything I could have done for myself. Her smile and the heartfelt tear as she told me how much she enjoyed our time together can't compare to any self-serving time I might have spent. Anyone who has ever helped another human being must know the satisfaction and good feeling that comes from helping someone. If you want to brighten a bad day or feel better about who you are, visit an elderly person to hear about their life, and I promise that you will both feel better when you leave than when you arrived. Just be sure to drop your drama at the door, or you may be thrown out!

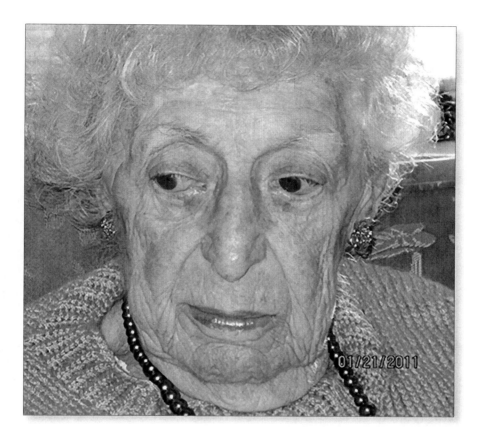

Caught in the system - Marie Harrison's Story

Marie Harrison was born on March 20, 1920, making her ninety-one at the time of this publication. I had not met Marie prior to the interview. A friend of mine who is the administrator of a local assisted-living facility asked a few residents if they would allow me to interview them for this book, and Marie agreed.

Marie was a bit uneasy when I went to her assisted-living apartment to interview her. She didn't know me from Adam and only went by what the administrator told her about me and my book project. My intention is to always be respectful and to make the interview as comfortable as if we were two friends chatting. Shortly into the interview, I could feel that Marie was more at ease, which was great because I didn't want her to feel uncomfortable or to feel regret in having agreed to meet with me. As you will understand through Marie's story, she has every reason to be cautious and careful about whom she trusts.

Marie was born and raised in Detroit, Michigan, one of six children. Her family lived in the country, which is now a suburb of Detroit. Her family had no running water and heated the home and well water with a wood-burning stove. Marie attended school, graduated, and attended a couple of years of community college, which was rare for women back then. Her childhood revolved around school and work for the family, which left little time for activities. She described doing laundry and cleaning for other families at thirteen to make one dollar a week, because her family didn't have much money. Work was passed down through her siblings, and because of their financial status, she described her family as "homebodies."

Marie described her parents as wonderful, saying, "They believed everyone should be working. They were very strict. We learned to wash clothes, iron, cook, clean, and my mom taught me to sew and knit," which became a passion of Marie's. Her family was Lutheran and the children were expected to attend church on Sundays. Sunday school at their church was an absolute must, according to Marie. As an adult, she taught Sunday school for seven years.

Marie's close friend throughout school was an African American girl. It was very rare in the 20s and 30s for a Caucasian girl and an African American girl to be best friends. Marie's friend was the only friend she talked about who was important to her in her school years. Marie wasn't allowed to date until she was eighteen years old, so she didn't do much dating and back then, kids weren't allowed to drive until they were eighteen.

Following high school and college, Marie went to work as an executive secretary for Ford Motor Company, where she remained for forty-two years. It was there she met her husband, Roger, who worked as an engineer for Ford. They started talking about marriage after six months of dating and married after one year together. Using the skills her mother taught her, Marie sewed her own wedding gown as well as the gowns of her six bridesmaids. Can you imagine? I don't know of a bride out there now who would even consider making her own wedding gown, let alone her bridesmaids' gowns.

Marie's greatest accomplishments, according to her, were the clothes she made for herself and others, and the more than thirty sweaters she knit. When I asked her why she didn't go on to be a designer, she said, "I don't like complaints." Sewing and knitting were enjoyable skills and her passion—something she could do for herself and for making gifts for her family and friends. She taught a few of the nurse's aides at her assisted-living facility how to knit. Marie seldom smiled during our discussion, but talking about her mother and the skills and passion she gave Marie sparked a fond and joyful expression.

Roger and Marie never had children. Marie needed to have a hysterectomy a year into their marriage. They weren't interested in adopting, so they spent their younger years working and golfing with friends they knew through their country club. Marie described the friendly competition and bantering between her husband and herself when they played golf. She recalled a hole-in-one that her husband made in which he remarked, "Now can you match that?" Strangely, that thought and remark were the only things that brought out a giggle and any evidence of joy in Marie. She talked a lot about their golf vacations and about going to Augusta to see Arnold Palmer and Jack Nicholson play in the Masters Tournament. Marie loves Tiger Woods but never had the opportunity to watch him in person. Her fondest and happiest times were with her husband; she loved the life they had together, which included lots of golf and friends.

Sometime around the year 2000, when Marie and Roger were approaching their fiftieth wedding anniversary, Roger left on a Sunday morning to take a drive, which he loved to do. Roger left around 9:00 a.m. and was still not home at 6:00 p.m., which was highly unusual. Finally, Marie received a phone call that Roger was seen partying more than an hour away from home at someone's home previously unknown to Roger or Marie. This was the first indication something was wrong and foretold a quick progression of memory loss.

They waited a few months for Roger to be evaluated, and by the time he was tested, he wasn't able to understand what was happening. Marie said she felt left out of the process because the physician didn't communicate or educate Marie about the testing and what he suspected was going on. The follow-up appointment for Roger's test results left Marie devastated. Marie described the doctor matter-of-factly telling her, "Your husband has dementia, try and make the best of it," and then he walked out of the room leaving Marie shocked and emotional. There was no concern, no support, no education, and no referrals for resources. No one came to her aid to console her as she sat there beside Roger, full of fear and emotions. Roger did not understand the news at this point, because the disease had progressed so quickly.

Can you imagine? "Make the best of it?" I don't think it gets colder than that! The crazy thing is, I have heard other stories similar to this one from patients and families I have met and cared for. With cancer, with terminal illness, and yes with Alzheimer's, there are doctors and healthcare professionals who have broken devastating news to patients and families as if the patient had a cold and should take an aspirin and get over it. Some people are clearly in the wrong profession!

After Marie took her husband home, she didn't seek any education, support, or help for her husband or herself. After coldly being told to deal with it, it's no wonder Marie didn't seek others in the profession. The pain of her husband's diagnosis was enough without the added disregard of her fear and feelings. There were no children to support Marie and Roger. They kept the dementia hidden from most of their friends and those they spent time with at the country club. They had an attorney who knew them well, and since Marie couldn't seek her husband's advice as she always had, she allowed the attorney to make decisions for her, which is now one of the biggest regrets of her life.

The attorney decided to put Roger in a nursing home soon after he was diagnosed. Because Marie did not want to be apart from her husband, she spent the following seven months living in the nursing home with him. She describes the care as horrible and told me how much she hated being there. Marie was married to Roger for fifty-one years before he passed away. After Marie lost Roger, she had only her attorney. She had lost contact with her friends and felt like he was the only one she could rely on to help her. The attorney convinced Marie to sell her home and car, and to move into an assisted living facility where she stayed for a year and a half. She didn't like the first facility and subsequently moved into the assisted living facility where I met her.

I was so sad to hear that while Marie was losing her love and best friend, she was being controlled by someone who never considered her wishes or feelings. Marie said, "I can never forgive him for putting Roger in that nursing home." Think about being in her place. The loneliness and fear she must have felt with no one to talk to, no one to understand, no one to support or help her through the worst time of her life. Marie continues to count on this attorney. She said, "I've known him for a long time, and I don't want to change now." She went on to say that she only consults with him when she has to. I can't imagine feeling like I had only one person to turn to in times of need, and it was someone that I disliked and didn't trust.

Marie's life now revolves around a little dog she rescued from a shelter. This dog appears to be all she has, even though she is surrounded by people and all the staff seem to love her. Her face exudes sadness. Marie no longer plays golf after falling and breaking both her hips, about a year apart, seven years ago. She doesn't drive, and she doesn't have family or any close friends.

I wonder how different things may have been had Marie and Roger had children, or a physician who cared, or an attorney who took Marie's feelings and preferences into consideration and supported her rather than controlled her. Can you see how much difference kindness, concern, support, and education could have made? Would those things have given her more happiness in the recent years? I can't imagine living an entire lifetime, then finding myself alone and wondering if anyone cares because I don't have any close family or friends.

Sadly, there are too many seniors sitting alone day after day without anyone investing any time or effort into making them feel loved and valued. As I look at Marie's photo and contemplate her story, I think I'll visit her this week and take her some flowers. It's not much but maybe, just maybe, I can give her a moment of love and a feeling of worth.

Marie's story is not exclusive. There are thousands of seniors out there who are alone, who have been misguided, and who are living lonely, depressed lives. Unfortunately, I think there will be more people like Marie in the future as more adults elect not to have children, or have fewer children, or have children who are spread all over the country and the world. In addition, our healthcare system is not focusing on geriatric training in medical and nursing schools.

There is discussion in the gay community about aging issues particular to their circumstances. The majority of gay individuals do not have children to assist them as they age, and many are shunned from senior living facilities and communities. Where are they to turn when care is needed? The debate is still strong regarding health insurance and other benefits for gay partners, so each is responsible for their own coverage. If you are a heterosexual believing this doesn't affect you, think again. The future and cost of care affects us all in one form or another.

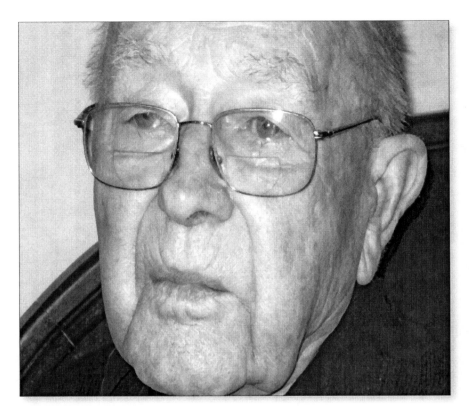

The life of a caregiver - Stan Smith's Story

Stan Smith is ninety-one years old. He was born on June 25, 1920, and grew up in California. Stan's father worked in research primarily dealing with citrus and insecticides to keep crops from being infested and damaged by bugs. Stan's dad must have had great influence in Stan's life and career path, because Stan became a researcher for the U.S. Department of the Interior and was a highly respected, highly sought-after specialist in aquatic ecology.

As with most men, Stan wanted to talk about his work more than anything else, and after hearing about the huge mark he made and the accomplishments he is credited with, it's easy to understand why his focus was on his work. Men tend to define themselves by their work anyway, so it took a lot of effort to change the subject in our interview in order to get more personal information from him.

Stan was highly involved in protecting the fishing industry in California in the 50s and 60s. The research and findings he reported to the Department of the Interior and to Congress were initially ignored, and the effects on the salmon industry and ecology of the waterways were taking a toll. Stan recognized that the dams which were being built to divert water to the southern California desert area during World War II were causing a loss of oxygen to the basin. The blue pike, once supported by a healthy ecosystem, were gone and Stan found the cause.

Dams continued to be built against his advice and began to take a bigger toll on the ecosystem that supported the salmon and fishing industry. The fishermen were angry and banded together to oppose the political decisions. The industry pressure caused Congress to finally take note of Stan's research and recommendations, and subsequently started removing the dams they spent so much time and money building.

Stan left California for Michigan to pursue research to support his efforts in California. He began making a name for himself as a highly respected and knowledgeable aquatic researcher while he was attending graduate school in Michigan. The government asked him to get involved in an investigation in the Great Lakes. The project was headed by three men: Stan, the man he worked for in California, and a mentor of Stan's who was legally blind. They were to investigate why fish in the Great Lakes were becoming extinct and to find out why there was a problem with parasites. A research vessel was built for the project but sat for two years without funding to operate it. Finally, after the project was idle for two years, funding became available and they gave Stan the vessel to dig deeper into the cause of the loss of fish.

In the mid 60s, Stan discovered the cause to be the dumping of raw sewage and industrial waste from Illinois into Lake Michigan, which in turn polluted Lake Erie. Reporters caught wind of Stan's findings and began announcing that Lake Erie was dead. This caused a huge boom in the sale of distilled water and was later credited as the influence for Earth Day. Stan later spent time doing research with Jacques Cousteau, and conducted research on all five Great Lakes.

By this time, Stan had been married for over twenty years to Anna, whom he met at Oregon State University and married in 1942. They had two children, a son and a daughter. During their lives, they were met with many health problems throughout their family. Anna took care of her sick mother who died an excruciating, painful death from a brain hemorrhage. Stan described his bride as an orphan at age twenty-one, because she had lost both of her parents. Stan noticed that Anna was less than social when they met and married, but he believed it was because she led a sheltered life caring for her parents. He thought if he could just get her out in the world, she would become social. As I listened to him, it seemed as if Stan took on the role of father figure, teacher, and protector from the time they met. He wanted to give Anna the life and care he thought she missed.

Their son, born in 1945, began exhibiting problems in first grade that caused enough concern to have him evaluated for psychological problems. He was diagnosed with "Schizophrenic Personality Disorder," Stan said. This isn't a true diagnostic category, but that was Stan's recollection at the time of our visit; it is possible their son was diagnosed with Childhood Onset Schizophrenia. Stan and Anna continued to have ongoing problems with their son throughout his school years. As he became an adult, he did not want to be away from his parents and on his own like most young adults. He wasn't able to hold a job or properly care for himself.

By the time their son was in his thirties, Stan had done everything possible to help him become independent. Stan and Anna's help didn't break his strong attachment to them, and they didn't know what else to do, so they retired and left for Australia. Stan felt they could force their son into independence by leaving, a drastic attempt to get their son to leave the nest. The fact that they felt they had to move so far away reveals the extent of their son's attachment and dependence.

While they were in Australia, they learned that their son was living in the car they had bought him. They stayed in Australia for two years and continued to try to help their son, but did not achieve the results they were hoping for. The next ten years brought one tragedy after another. Stan cared for his mother, aunt, son, and in many ways, his wife Anna. Stan wrote letters to his mom and aunt when he traveled. Stan was on a trip to Mexico when he got news that his mom died. Stan's mother died in her bed holding one of two letters he had sent her. The first letter was opened and in her hand, and the second lay next to her unopened. By a strange coincidence, his aunt died not much later, also holding a letter Stan had written her. By Stan's report, all the women in his life were highly dependent on him. His mom, aunt, and wife all relied on him for support and assistance, as did his son.

One day in the early 90s, Stan was watching television. A report was on about Asperger's syndrome. Stan felt this was exactly what was affecting his wife and son. He did a lot of research, as researchers do, and is convinced that they both suffered from this illness. This was the cause of their social inability, dependence, and strange characteristics associated with this syndrome, according to Stan.

Stan's life was a combination of tragedy and success. Stan has been a caregiver his entire life. He has gone through some of his own health problems and an injury that caused big changes in his life. Nearly four years ago, Stan injured himself while cutting a tree down. He fell and fractured his pelvis. That injury caused him to move to the assisted living facility he and Anna now reside in.

Stan has a serious heart condition, which he refrained from naming. When he and Anna were still living in their home, Stan didn't feel well one evening after dinner and went to lie down. He then experienced a horrible pain, "like an elephant sitting on my chest." As a nurse, I knew this meant he had a heart attack. He said, "All of a sudden, everything turned black and then suddenly changed to the most beautiful pearly radiating glow. I was above my body like I was drifting. I could see Anna in the kitchen doing dishes and cleaning the kitchen. It was as if the wall was translucent; I could see and hear everything. The next thing I knew, Anna came in and woke me up. My pillow was soaked." Stan said that experience changed his personality. He described himself as rather strict and hard. "Probably too hard," by his own admission. "Now," he says, "I have feelings and patience for people like I never did before."

You may be thinking this was a spiritual experience, as I did. I was rather shocked that Stan revealed to me that he doesn't believe in God. He grew up going to Sunday school and church. He didn't state a specific time or event that caused him to believe that God doesn't exist.

Anna now has Alzheimer's and is in the severe stages of the disease. Stan is her full-time primary caregiver. He tries to keep her active, and every night he reads her the journals she'd written over the course of her life. He wonders what will happen to her if he dies before she does.

What I took away from my interview with Stan was twofold. I found him to be an incredible man of strength and fortitude with a deep love and loyalty to the people in his life. He is highly intelligent and made great contributions to our ecology and society. On the other hand, I find his life and story to be very sad. I can't psychoanalyze Stan or his own evaluation of his life, the spiritual experience I believe he had, or why he is at a place in time when his life is limited and he is not concerned about his death. No matter what I think or you think about his life and beliefs, Stan declared, "I have had the happiest life, and I wouldn't change a thing."

What will constitute your happiness when you face your last years? Will it be family, contributions to our society, memories, or contentment, no matter what you go through? Of course, we don't know the answers until we get there, but it's definitely worth thinking about on the way. Maybe the lessons are to care for the people you love and do everything you can while you are able.

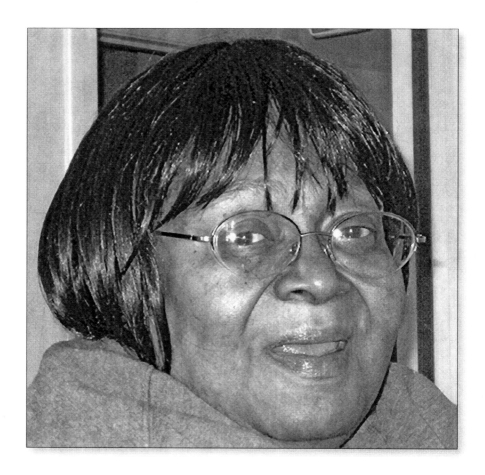

Senior living isn't just for seniors - Emily Baker's Story

Emily Baker was born in Chicago on June 13, 1947. Emily is sixty-four years old and doesn't yet meet the sixty-five-or-older Social Security criterion for a senior. I interviewed Emily and included her in this book because she has lived in an assisted living facility for the past three years. Emily's story illustrates that you don't have to be classified as a senior to find yourself in need of care and living a senior lifestyle.

There are people in their twenties, thirties, forties, and fifties who are living in nursing homes among those who are sixty-five years and older. I have met and cared for younger individuals who have been forced to live in nursing homes among the elderly because of debilitating diseases that could not, or would not, allow them to remain home or with family. In 2005, Emily suffered severe mental and physical injuries when a bus she was riding in was hit by a truck and she flew out of the back window. The injuries she suffered were the cause of her early entry into the world normally reserved for seniors.

Emily had an extremely difficult and tragic life, yet she managed to come through it all with an amazing attitude and perspective. I was surprised at how open Emily was in revealing the tragedies of her life, since we hadn't met prior to the interview. She was very pleasant, even joyful, despite our discussion of her past and the things she had gone through.

Emily grew up in the home of her mother and the man she believed to be her father in the projects of Chicago. Her father was physically abusive to her mother and to her. She took beatings for her three sisters because she felt she could handle it better than her sisters could. Therefore, Emily and her mom were the targets of his anger and abuse. Her father was a professional boxer, which gives us some idea of his strength.

When Emily was growing up, people often asked her if the man she knew as her dad was indeed her father. Emily didn't inquire about this until she was an adult. When she did ask this man if he was her father, his response was, "Go ask your mother." Emily never knew the real truth, but she feels like he wasn't her biological father.

Emily's perspective towards this man and the abuse she suffered at his hands is very forgiving. When Emily talked about him, she stated, "He couldn't help it; he was beaten at the age of five because he didn't bring in as much cotton as his brother did." She went on to say that her dad ran away from home at fourteen and ate out of garbage cans. Emily always puts her food scraps in individual plastic bags which she throws into the garbage, so if any-one who is hungry picks through her trash, they will be given more dignity. This simple act reveals her ability to love, understand, and forgive a man that caused her so much pain and was not even believed to be her father.

Emily married at eighteen so she could escape the abuse and dysfunction in her family. She wanted to join the military, but her mother convinced her not to by claiming, "Women in the army are all lesbians." The home environment was so bad, Emily would have accepted any proposal be-cause she was so desperate to escape.

The abuse didn't just come at the hands of this man she thought was her father. She was raped by her uncle at the age of ten and told me, "I was raped so much, I felt like I was in *The Color Purple*." A very strong and sad statement, for sure. As is common with young girls who experience sexual abuse, Emily looked for her worth by offering her body in a desire to be loved and became pregnant at fifteen. She had four children with a cheating husband who also impregnated another woman, which was something her father had done to her mother.

Amid the negative environment and influences, Emily found solace in art. She attended craft classes and volunteered at local nursing homes and youth programs to teach what she learned and loved. Her talent didn't go unrecognized, and she was awarded an art scholarship for college. Sadly, she gave it up to marry so she could escape the home environment she lived in. She now helps residents with crafts in the activities department of the assisted living facility that is her home.

Emily is extremely proud of her eight grandchildren and one great-grand-child. She has one daughter who lives nearby; her other three children live out of state. Emily's ten-year-old niece is another source of pride and joy. She sings and plays instruments, and was scheduled to entertain the residents in the week following my interview.

As in all interviews, I asked Emily what her best advice was. She elaborated more than most, giving me several bits of wisdom. She said, "Trust yourself and your judgement as much as you can. Never say you can't do it, because you don't know what you're capable of. Forgive others, because you also will need forgiveness. You never know what you'd do in the same circumstance, and everyone makes mistakes." Emily continued, "Accept your own shortcomings and others. If you live to see another day, you can start all over again." Emily finished by telling me she was grateful she lived through all the difficulties adding, "Some couldn't."

I left the interview feeling sad and inspired. I am sad for the many physical and emotional things that Emily had gone through but amazed and inspired by her strength, forgiveness, and attitude. I am grateful to Emily that she allowed me and you to know about the deep wounds and strength within her, and that she trusted me and the intentions of this book.

I think about the people who meet and care for Emily. I wonder if they give her the love and kindness that she deserves and has lacked so much. Unless you make an effort to spend time with people like Emily and the millions residing in assisted living and nursing home facilities, you might not be sensitive to their hurts and needs. Do you think care providers would offer additional love, attention, kindness, and respect if they knew how much Emily had been through? I believe they would. It is important to take the time to understand that every person has a past life of hurts, emotions, tragedies, and needs. Whether we have the time to learn about them or not, they all deserve kindness, recognition, respect, and dignified, attentive treatment and care.

Would you want to add additional pain to Emily's life? Do you think there have been healthcare workers and professionals who weren't sensitive to Emily's need for love and value, and who directly or indirectly added to her wounds of the past? I would almost bet there has been. Too many care providers never consider the feelings and needs of their patients outside of the physical ailment they may be attending to. Too many care providers are focused on themselves or the task at hand, and don't consider their attitude, approach, and the whole health of the patient. Disregard for the care recipient's thoughts and feelings can cause more harm when you don't know their history.

Degrees and classes do not make a great care provider. Great care providers have knowledge and empathy; they instinctively consider the thoughts and feelings of their patients and tend to those as much as the physical care tasks at hand.

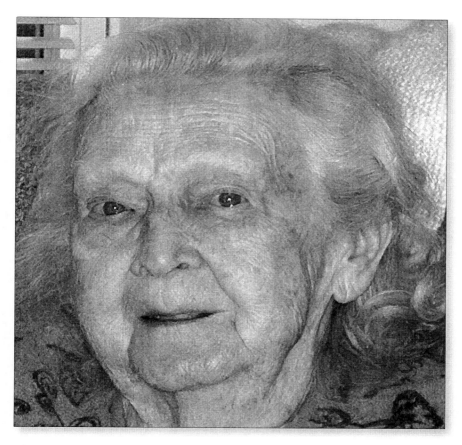

The storehouse of the dying - Inez Mason's Story

Inez Mason was nearing her ninety-fourth birthday when I interviewed her. She was born February 2, 1919. At ninety-two, you might expect a frail, quiet woman at peace in this time of her life, but you haven't met Inez! She is a rebellious powerhouse with strong opinions and convictions. Inez is a highly accomplished and intelligent woman who still has plans for the future.

Inez was a biochemistry professor and researcher whose life began in Illinois. Being a science major and entering a career in biochemistry was extremely rare for women in the 1940s. Inez worked during World War

II as an inspector in food factories for what she called "war food." Many women worked in factories at that time, because our country needed them to support the war effort, but few held such prestigious positions.

Our discussion focused more on her life as an adult than as a child, and much of it pertained to her work and career. Her appreciation of her own intelligence, work, and contributions in biochemistry didn't come early in her life. Keep in mind that women were second to men at that time. It was expected that women would marry, raise families, and support their husbands' careers and ambitions. Women worked during the war to support the men and were not seen as career women.

Inez was different because she was going to do it all. She married a navy man who was a chemical engineer, and they divorced twenty-three years ago. They adopted two daughters because Inez wasn't able to have children. She spoke with great pride about her daughters, including the fact that one of her daughters was a planner for the 1996 Olympics held in Atlanta, Georgia.

Inez is the last living child of eight. All her friends are dead. That is a lot of loss. Imagine having seven brothers and sisters and losing them all. Imagine living longer than anyone who was close to you and being without any siblings, parents, or friends. Her brother, Bill, was one of her toughest losses. He died of brain cancer, and Inez misses relying on him. She said, "I went to Bill for everything." She went on to say, "Losing everybody makes me feel like a lonely dinosaur."

Despite all her losses, Inez said her divorce was the worst time of her life, because she didn't see it coming. In some ways, it was also the best thing for Inez, because she finally could recognize her accomplishments. She was an accomplished researcher biochemistry professor at the prestigious University of Michigan and had her name on a medication patent. In addition, Inez spent a lot of time volunteering for worthy causes such as

Alzheimer's, a local hospice agency, and the Ronald McDonald House in Ann Arbor, Michigan.

Inez has not been able to continue her volunteer work because she has gone through one illness and injury after another. She was stricken with colon cancer that required surgery and subsequent colostomy and feeding tube, suffered a fractured hip from a fall, and is now losing her vision to macular degeneration. These events collectively led to her loss of independence and move into assisted living, which she describes as "a storehouse for people waiting to die." Inez had difficulty finding a place that would accept her because of her colostomy and feeding tube. She believes it takes too much time for the nurses, and that's why many places wouldn't accept her.

I think the general public believes that long-term care facilities accept anyone with the finances and a desire to live there; that is not the case at all. Medical conditions, mobility, and psychiatric illnesses are all causes of rejection. If you were in Inez's shoes, how would you feel if you lost everyone who meant something to you, went through cancer and a radical surgery, and was forced into a care facility because of physical decline, only to be rejected by a facility because of the results of cancer which were not in your control?

Inez didn't choose cancer. She didn't choose loss of independence, and she hates to rely on anyone for assistance. She has lost the ability to do the things that she enjoyed and that brought value to her life. These days bring little enjoyment for Inez. Even though she lives in a very nice assisted living facility, she dislikes being there so much that she has not made friends, vested herself in activities, or accepted her loss of independence. She yearns for her once active and productive life and to contribute again to society.

Do you think that Inez would enjoy her life more if the people around her—and we, as a society—recognized, appreciated, and utilized her contributions, skills, knowledge, and talent? Inez is a very sharp, intelligent woman. She needs to feel valued, and we are not meeting her needs. Don't you suppose there is something Inez could still do to be productive and feel valued? Her knowledge of and experience in biochemistry could be shared with university students who need research for term papers or tutoring. With her volunteer experience and the knowledge and understanding she gained from working with patients with Alzheimer's, terminal illness, and families of sick children, she could provide occasional support to those struggling in these areas.

If we just spent time with people like Inez to learn about their lives and the experience and lessons they have to share, they would feel valued. When people sit in a long term-care facility day after day feeling like they are being housed for death rather than used for life, it's no wonder the rate of depression is so high among them.

When I asked Inez what she wanted to pass along, she said, "Do everything while you can." I also asked her what she wants people to know about her. She responded, "I hope people know that I was easy to get along with, I was interested in other people's lives, and I spent time contributing." I summarize that as being valued.

When I asked seniors about lessons they want to share or what each person wants us to know about them, they never talk about anything materialistic. It's never about the money earned, the houses purchased, or how clean their house was. It's never about the hours put into a career. It is always about relationships and contribution. It seems to come down to two things: did I treat people well, and did I serve? Those are the important things to keep in mind as we go through our lives, because we all will ask ourselves those same questions. Our answers will come with regret or satisfaction. Unless you die early or unexpectedly, there will come a day when you will no longer be able to do the things you wanted to or thought you would do. "Someday" will be gone. "One of these days" will not come.

If all Inez left for us was the knowledge that it's all about loving and serving, we couldn't ask for a better contribution, but she has and can contribute so much more.

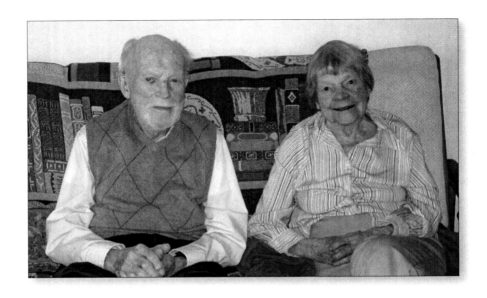

Fred and Janet Howard - A love story

Fred and Janet Howard are the oldest married couple I can recall ever meeting. Fred just passed his 101st birthday, and Janet is approaching her 98th birthday. Janet was born April 18, 1914, and Fred was born December 9, 1910. They have been married for seventy-one years—they married a couple weeks before the attack on Pearl Harbor in 1941.

Their early love story is documented in a book titled *Whistle While You Wait*. It is a compilation of Fred's and Janet's letters as a newlywed couple separated during World War II. The book reads like fine poetry and is very telling of the time and language of two young people in love in the early to mid twentieth century.

When I went to interview the Howards, I knew only their names and ages. I had no idea who I was going to meet and what I would learn about these wonderful people. I interviewed Fred as Janet sat quietly nearby, unable to appropriately respond because of the dementia that took her memories.

Fred and Janet lived in Chicago prior to Fred's being drafted into the war. Fred was enlisted as an officer bombardier in the Army Air Corps two years after going to a secret bomb-site school. Fred flew fifty-seven combat missions, jumped out of his B-25 plane at the foot of Mount Etna in Italy, and lost a good friend who was taken as a POW. Those are a few examples from a long list of experiences and accomplishments during Fred's service to our country. Fred's tour of duty just preceded the timing of Joseph Heller's novel, *Catch 22*, which drew upon Heller's experiences as a B-25 bombardier and could have easily included Fred's experiences, too.

As similar as Fred and Joseph Heller's military services were, their careers followed a similar post-war path. While Fred was in the war, Janet and their first child moved to Garrett Park, Maryland, which is twelve miles from the White House. Janet purchased a Chevy House which came with a Murphy bed, an Atwater Kent radio, and a Chevy automobile in the garage. I thought Fred was kidding when he told me this, but he was not. It is another bit of knowledge I gained through time with someone who lived so long ago.

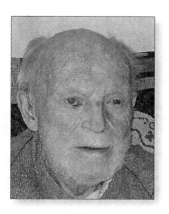

When Fred returned from war, he got a job at the Library of Congress. In 1928, prior to his time in the Army, Fred won a writing competition that provided a four-year college scholarship. He wanted to be an actor, but he chuckled as said he was "awful!" Fred's dad wanted him to be an inventor, and he dabbled in trying to invent headlights that turned with the steering wheel of the car, but he lost everything and his future as an inventor. Fred returned to research and writing, in which he excelled.

Fred worked with Fred Praeger as an editor. Not knowing anything about Praeger or Praeger Publishing, I didn't know where the conversation was going or why this publisher stood out in Fred's career. As the conversation continued, Fred told of the controversy Praeger elicited. Praeger was an Austrian intelligence officer and military official in Europe during World War II. He sought communist dissidents from the Soviet Union, East Germany, Czechoslovakia, and Hungary during the height of the Cold War and brought the realities of communism to readers in the U.S. His activities were suspect for the CIA and caused an investigation into Praeger. The controversy was too much, so he fled the U.S.

Praeger was fortunate enough to come to the U.S. in 1938, but his family wasn't as fortunate. They died in Auschwitz. Imagine being the editor of those manuscripts. Here I was, sitting with Fred Howard, an accomplished war hero and copy editor who worked for the Library of Congress. He worked as an editor on some of the most controversial writings of our time and even worked for the Smithsonian, which in itself was fascinating. Fred was not finished surprising me.

In 1972, Fred wrote and published his first novel, titled *Charlie Flowers and the Melody Gardens*, about a boy named Charlie Flowers who lived in Chicago between wars. Charlie lost his parents and lived with his grandmother whose boarding house overlooked Melody Gardens and the magical things that the garden brought. Fred was sixty-two when his novel was finally published. If that isn't enough, get ready for more.

As I mentioned, Fred worked for the Library of Congress and the Smithsonian. He worked there at just the right time to be one of the individuals presented with the original letters and technical papers of the Wright Brothers, which Orville willed to the Library of Congress upon his death in 1948. Orville stipulated in his will that the documents were to be

shared with the public. Those same documents now sit in the Smithsonian Institute in the archives of the National Air and Space Museum.

Fred subsequently wrote and published *Wilbur and Orville: a Biography of
the Wright Brothers* in 1987 at the age of seventy-seven. There are several
versions of Fred's book on the Wright Brothers, and Fred allowed me to
photograph the covers of all the versions in his possession, as well as his
other two books. Many books have been written about the Wright Brothers, but how many of them are by an author who actually handled and
read their original technical papers? I felt as if I was one degree away from
the Wright Brothers themselves as I listened to Fred. What a privilege!

When I went to meet and interview Fred and Janet Howard, I had no idea
what I would hear, who they would be, or that I would be sitting with
someone so accomplished. Did I ever expect to sit with someone who
had the original Wright Brothers papers in their hands, or who flew fifty-
seven combat missions for our protection and freedom? No, I sure didn't,
but I left Fred and Janet's small apartment that day knowing more about
our nation's history, more about the world of publishing and historical
archives, and with a copy of Fred's novel, which I asked him to sign. I felt
overwhelmingly honored when Fred gave me a copy of his book. I felt
privileged to have met Fred and Janet, and to have heard about their lives
and experiences.

Since that interview, I found a copy of *Whistle While You Wait* and re-
visited Fred and Janet to bring some treats and ask for his autograph on
the book of letters between them. At 101 and nearly 98, I don't know
how much longer these two wonderful people will be with us, but I hope
someone else cares enough to spend time with them and has the privilege
of hearing their story, because it is an honor that will stay with me for a
very long time.

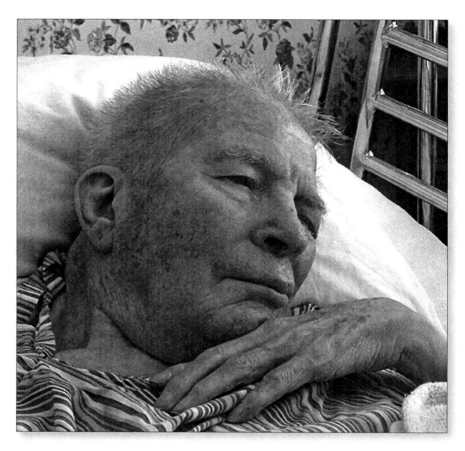

Carlton Houghtalin - My inspiration and friend

Carlton's story was in Part 1 of the book, but I wanted to include his photo here. This was Carlton in bed at his niece Susan's home. He didn't talk much anymore when I took this photo, but he was very aware of everything going on around him. I wonder what his thoughts were at this time when he was in need of full care.

Carlton served our country in the military. He and his wife provided time, love, and care for their nieces and for their foster children and adopted children. Carlton gave his life for the betterment of others, and I hope he knew how special he was as he lay in bed so quietly. Carlton's contribution is not finished, even though he has left us. He was the inspiration for this book and will in many ways be a huge part of anyone's receiving better treatment and care because of this book. I hope he knows that.

Chapter 6
More Behind the Old Face

Throughout my career, I have met and spent time with many different people from construction workers to master sculptors, from stay-at-home mothers to missionaries. They all enhanced my life in some way.

Mary Pickett - Pillar of strength

One lady I often think about is Mary Pickett. Mary had one of the most incredible stories of strength I've ever heard, yet she wondered why on earth I would be interested in her life and story. Mary was born October 9, 1910. I met her through her granddaughter, whom I knew through networking. I mentioned I was interviewing seniors for this book, and she told me her grandmother was the strongest lady she knew and thought I'd be interested in her story.

I met Mary in a local nursing home. She was a petite lady with visible scarring on her face and hands. She was soft spoken and a bit shy when the interview started, but as we talked she relaxed and we had a wonderful visit!

Mary was born in Detroit and had a grandmother in Canada. Her parents took Mary on a boat to Canada on the weekends to visit. When Mary was visiting her grandmother at the age of two and a half, she went through a tragedy unlike anything our generation can fathom.

In 1912, her grandmother did not have electricity, so their source of light came from kerosene lanterns. Somehow, in the night, Mary knocked the lit lantern over and she was covered in burning oil. The thought of a toddler burning is horrific enough, but to hear Mary describe the months following gave me insight into her incredible strength.

You see, this happened to Mary before World War I. There weren't hospitals in every city or public hospitals as we know them today. There was nowhere to take this severely burned toddler. There weren't medications and treatments to help her. All of us have experienced burns to one degree or another, and even the slightest burn can cause days of pain, so imagine flaming oil stuck to your skin like adhesive on a stamp. Imagine the screams of a child and the family who witnessed that nightmare. Imagine not having a hospital to go to. Those of us who grew up in modern society never consider how emergencies were handled before hospitals and healthcare existed. Mary's story was an eye-opening experience as I looked at the scars on her face and wondered how she lived through the pain.

Mary's grandmother lived across the street from a doctor, and for the next few months Mary recovered in bed at her grandmother's house with care from her family and the doctor. There were no pain medications to give Mary, but the doctor had an amazing intelligence and heart. He washed Mary's burns in saline solution and took a risk that his peers and locals thought was crazy. This incredible doctor cut skin from his own body to graft onto Mary's face. This was a procedure well before its time. It is truly a miracle that Mary didn't die of infection. Antibiotics were not developed at that time. The first cure from penicillin, which was the first antibiotic developed, didn't occur until 1930.

It took years for Mary to fully recover. As a child bound to her bed, she lost her ability to walk. So much of the growth and abilities she had gained by age two and a half were lost. There was a very lengthy rehabilitation process besides the recovery from the actual burns. Emotionally, I am not sure Mary has ever fully recovered. She talked about her hair growing back and waiting until she looked normal enough to go to school. She told me about the teasing from the other children. She distinctly remembered a boy named Stanley who tormented Mary with name-calling and teasing from age six to twelve. Evidence of the emotional scars from the bullying lies in the fact that nearly one hundred years later, Mary recalls the bully's name and how much pain he caused her.

If this tragedy wasn't enough, Mary ended up a single mother of eight children, left by an abusive alcoholic husband. She watched three sons go off to World War II at the same time, and worked extremely hard as a nurse's aide to support her family. Mary wanted to be a nurse but was denied by the school because they said she wasn't strong enough. Mary would beg to differ, and I have to agree with her!

Our conversation also included times and things in Mary's life that brought her joy, which was evident in her beautiful smile and eyes. She loved playing outdoors as a child and especially liked ice skating and swimming. Mary's fondest memories revolved around her parents, siblings, and children. Her father always talked about wanting a large family, but her parents were only able to have four children, so in many ways it seems like Mary fulfilled her father's dream by raising eight children, which is her proudest accomplishment.

Now you can see why Mary was one of the strongest women I've ever met. Mary's story isn't famous. She didn't make headlines or leave some newsworthy or notable contribution to society, but her story is no less important. The lessons we learn are often more important to our lives than the inventions we use. If you want to know how to get through tough times, go spend time with Mary! If you want to know how to have more joy in your life or how to live well, take time to hear the life histories of seniors in your neighborhood, in a long-term care facility, or in your church.

When I left Mary that day, I'm not sure who was more grateful. She took my hand, looked me in the eyes, and said, "I enjoyed your visit so much, thank you for coming, and feel free to come visit me any time." Do you know what Mary was grateful for? She was grateful that someone outside of her family cared. She was grateful to have a long and enjoyable visit and conversation. She was grateful to relive her days of ice skating on the pond and summers splashing in the lake. For a brief time, Mary was young again. I could see it in her eyes and hear it in her voice. I was privileged to go on that journey with her.

To give you a little more insight into people I've met and had the privilege of getting to know, I'll share a few more experiences. When I worked as a home health and hospice nurse or went out to hospitals and nursing homes to assess or care for a patient, I knew very little about them. I'd have a name, address, some basic information and a diagnosis or description of their care needs. It is only through meeting them and asking about them that I understood who I was going to help. Because my main purpose was to address their health or care needs, I didn't always get to know much more about them.

As a homecare agency owner, my assessments were a bit different. Besides addressing the health and care needs, I also included in my assessments questions about occupation previous to retirement, hobbies, interests, their life history, and preferences. I believe it's important to the overall care of the patient to know more about them and their lives in order to provide a basis for the caregiver to better understand who they will be caring for and how to initiate conversation regarding their interests. As healthcare providers we are treating people with a medical condition, not a medical condition in and of itself. The patient is not the condition, and the more we realize that, the better our care giving will be.

Charles Singer-The Incredible Artist

A few years ago, I was called to assist a gentleman, Charles Singer, who was just released from the hospital. When I arrived at his home, I was greeted by his daughter who apologized for not being ready and escorted me to the living room while she helped her parents finish up lunch. I waited patiently, looking around at the amazing sculptures they had in their home. I assumed they were collectors and complimented them on their sculptures, especially a bronze sculpture, beautifully detailed, of a little boy with a much larger angel looking over him. It stood about two feet tall. Charles' daughter revealed that her dad was a master sculptor.

Charley, as he preferred to be called, was humble about his incredible artistic ability. The statue that I was so drawn to was a small model version of a much larger sculpture that sits at the grave of a son they lost as a little boy. They went on to tell me that Charley created bronze sculptures that sit in front of government buildings and in museums. This incredible artist was still sculpting at ninety! He told me, "It takes me a bit longer these days." I was more impressed that he was still sculpting!

Lucille Porter- True to her heritage

Another patient of mine was Lucille Porter. She was a sweet but stubborn African American woman whom I also visited in her home as she was beginning her post-hospital recovery. She started the African American festival in Ann Arbor and proudly displayed her credits and articles on the wall next to the worn-out recliner she spent her days in. She spoke of her concerns about the future of her festivals and how she disliked sagging pants and rap songs. She was quite a character, and I loved spending time with her.

Margaret Overbee- A simple trip to church

I had a sweet, tiny patient in my earlier years as a homecare nurse who followed me from job to job. She had a tracheotomy and feeding tube, a result of rheumatoid arthritis that crippled and mangled her body so much she could barely breathe and couldn't walk or use her hands very well. I loved that little lady. Her name was Margaret. She had frequent hospitalizations and exacerbations of respiratory problems, so she was on and off home care. We bonded well the first time I cared for her. I'd help get her well enough to discharge her, and she'd need us again a few months later. She liked me so she requested me as her nurse every time she needed home health care. At one point, I left a particular job and she somehow found out what company I went to. She followed me, requesting me and only me as her nurse.

Margaret had a live-in caregiver from another company who, I realized over time, was less than compassionate. Some days, I would visit Margaret and she would cry about her life, being stuck in that house, and the lack of kind and compassionate care. One problem was that the live-in caregiver would be there literally months at a time with no time off. That type of responsibility is difficult for a family member let alone an employee who never has time for themselves or their own life and family. No doubt she was burned out, but it was not Margaret's fault, it was the fault of the agency. Yet, Margaret paid the price.

Many times, I would visit when Margaret was watching TV-evangelist

Benny Hinn, so I knew she was a Christian. One day, as Margaret sat with me crying about her life, or lack thereof, I asked, "If you could go anywhere, where would you want to go?" She said, "Church."

Margaret had one living relative who was involved in her care—a niece who lived out of town. I told Margaret if I could get permission from her niece and the agency I worked for, I would take her to church. I didn't anticipate that would cause her to cry harder, but it did. I'm not sure if she cried harder because there was hope of getting out of that house she felt imprisoned in, because I cared enough to want to take her out, or because of the possibility of going to church, but she cried happy tears for the first time.

Since Margaret was an African American woman and I had seen Benny Hinn on her TV, I thought that my church may not suit her needs. I talked to a couple of my African American friends, and they suggested I bring Margaret to their church where one of my friends sang in the choir. I got the permission I needed to take Margaret and spoke to her live-in caregiver to prepare Margaret and herself to go to church the next Sunday.

That day sticks out as one of my happiest memories! Margaret couldn't have been happier or more grateful. The members of the church took an immediate liking to her; several prayed with her and over her as Margaret cried tears of joy. I am not telling you this story to brag or present myself as some type of martyr. I am telling you this because this simple effort of taking a couple hours out of my life brought Margaret more joy than she'd had in years! The blessing was really mine. To do something so simple that can make such a difference in someone's life is a true joy and blessing. If you want to bring happiness to your own life, take time to bring joy to a senior. That day will always be in my heart as a happy day! I can easily recall the joy on Margaret's face with that adorable smile she had.

Unfortunately, Margaret died when I was on vacation, so I never got the chance to say goodbye or pay my respects, but memories of Margaret and the time we spent together will be with me for life. I still miss seeing her and the bright smile she had when I visited.

When I set out to write this book and interview seniors for it, I had no agenda. I only wanted to provide a basis for understanding so you could see there is more *Behind the Old Face* and help you understand what it's like to be in the shoes of your parents, grandparents, neighbors, the old couple in line at the store, the lady in the wheelchair at the doctor's office, and the person you are feeding in the nursing home. I knew a couple of the seniors featured in this book before the actual interview, but many I did not.

I am sure it wasn't easy for them to allow a stranger to come in asking the details of their lives and inquiring into their thoughts and feelings. As much as I have worked with seniors—I have literally met and cared for thousands— I still learned things I never expected, felt more compassion and inspiration than before I met them, and will carry their impression in my heart. I am very grateful and honored they were all willing to share themselves and the secrets and feelings of their lives with me and for this book, and you should be grateful too. These individuals live in my neighborhood and without this book, I would have never had the privilege to meet or know about them.

Who is living in your neighborhood? Who has lost the ability to walk, or paint, or teach, or do surgery and lives nearby in the local nursing home? Who are we ignoring and dismissing because their face and abilities have aged? Who is lonely and neglected, and even abused, who may have fought for our freedom, saved a child, or invented a product you are currently using? Where will you be in twenty, thirty, or forty years? Will you be the lonely dependant woman in a wheelchair hoping for someone to care, or the man alone day after day without a phone call or visitor, or the person whose family and friends have all died as you sit wondering how long you have left to live?

Life as an aging adult doesn't have to be lonely, depressing, or lost. There are answers and choices to enhance life for seniors. There are ways to reduce loneliness and depression, provide value, and help them remain at home no matter how much care they may need or how much income they have. There are ways to keep people engaged and not make them feel like a burden when their physical bodies or minds fail.

I have seen more advocacy for an animal than an abused senior. Does that make any sense? We support Toys for Tots, the local animal shelter, and a host of other programs, yet who is supporting the seniors who are without their own socks or undergarments in Medicaid nursing homes? Who is helping seniors pay for the medications they cannot afford and forgo to pay for food? Who is helping the elderly veteran who is on the street, homeless? Who cares if lonely seniors spend holidays alone and never receive a birthday or Christmas gift? Do they not deserve as much as an animal or as a child without a toy at Christmas?

Part 3 of this book provides answers, but before you read on, take the time to ask yourself what kind of life you'll want when you are eighty or ninety? Can you see yourself in any of the seniors you met in these pages? Have you had a family member who was treated poorly in the hospital or a living facility? Have you been less than kind and respectful to a patient or witness a co-worker disrespecting a patient? Folks, this happens every single day to thousands of seniors.

Do you have a different perspective than you did when you opened the book? I hope that you will think differently when you come in contact with and care for an aging adult. I hope you understand how much you can mean to their lives, how much they need and deserve to be treated with respect, dignity, kindness, and compassion, and how much they still have to offer.

I hope you will take the time to brighten a senior's day, learn more from them, and involve yourself in advocacy for their better treatment, living, and care.

Part 3   The Future of Aging

Chapter 7
Vision for the Coming Elder Boom
The need for change

After reading Parts 1 and 2, I suspect you see a need for change even if you didn't before you started the book. If you already knew we need a better system for providing care for aging adults, this book has probably given you a reminder or more reasons why our current system is ineffective and substandard, now and for the future.

In thinking about the causes and possible solutions to our current problems, we have to break down what the problems are first. In a summary, we know from Chapter 4 that we are facing unprecedented growth in the aging population, so the problems we currently have will increase if we don't come up with solutions.

We have social, psychological, and financial problems, and we have demographic and housing problems. Those problems apply to the elderly population and the population at large. There is currently a shortage of professional caregivers, nurses, geriatric physicians, physician assistants, and nurse practitioners. The nursing industry has been working on recruitment and incentives for years now but isn't any closer to solving the shortage, especially as our population begins the shift into aging.

There has been a propensity for nurses in other areas of nursing to disregard geriatric nurses as less capable than "real nurses." Where does this come from? Geriatric nurses specialize just like pediatric nurses special-ize, yet they are viewed differently by their own peers. This bias is also contributing to a shortage in the area of geriatric nursing. Physicians want to specialize in elite areas of medicine like trauma, surgery, cardiology, and neurology, but few specialize in geriatric medicine. The uninformed perspective and attitudes within our own field is detrimental to the future of medicine and healthcare.

The needs are much greater for caregivers and nurses aides than for nurses and physicians, because most seniors need the nonmedical assistance and care to maintain their independence and remain safe. The pay is low for caregivers and nurses aides, and the work can be very difficult. Even for those who love the elderly and this work, the retention rate is low because other professions pay higher wages or offer health insurance, which is also rare in this work. So what can we do to solve this problem and encourage more people to desire this profession? There must be incentives to help encourage and retain great care providers. There are ways to help solve this problem, too.

Chapter 8
The Time for Action

Anyone who wants to improve something has a vision. Vision is what makes things happen and society progress, and that is why companies, organizations, foundations, and most groups have vision statements. Every leadership training includes writing a vision statement.

Maybe you will recognize some of these popular quotes on vision:
The empires of the future are empires of the mind.
— **Winston Churchill**

Where there is no vision the people perish.
— **Proverbs 29:18**

Dream lofty dreams, and as you dream, so shall you become.
Your Vision is the promise of what you shall one day be.
Your Ideal is the prophecy of what you shall at last unveil.
— **James Allen**

Vision without a task is only a dream. A task without a vision is but drudgery. But vision with a task is a dream fulfilled.
— **Anonymous**

Big thinking precedes great achievement.
— **Wilferd Peterson**

Dissatisfaction and discouragement are not caused by
the absence of things but the absence of vision.
— **Anonymous**

The most pathetic person in the world is someone
who has sight but has no vision.
— **Helen Keller**

A vision is not just a picture of what could be;
it is an appeal to our better selves, a call to become something more.
— **Rosabeth Moss Kanter**

As you can see by these eight quotes about vision, nothing is accomplished, improved, or successful without it!

I have asked many people if they thought we needed improvements in senior care, and to no surprise, one hundred percent said yes. What is a surprise is that one hundred percent didn't have any concrete thoughts or ideas on how to improve it. There is a lack of vision.

After thirty plus years in senior care and advocacy, I feel it's time for the vision. It is time for concrete answers to solve current problems, reduce healthcare costs, and improve the quality of life for some of the most deserving people on the planet! It's time to divert the impending crisis and make things happen!

My vision is concrete, realistic, and very doable. It solves problems, reduces costs, and improves the quality of life for aging adults. After spending over thirty years with aging adults, family caregivers, and healthcare workers and professionals, in every type of living situation available today, I can say my vision developed out of the trenches of eldercare. This book didn't start with any thoughts of including a particular way of living, and was only intended to draw empathy to improve care, but when my publisher asked me to put on paper my vision for how I think life would be better for the elderly, we both got excited! With that said, here is my vision.

I see a society that values its elders and understands the changes and challenges we encounter as we age. We all have our life story, thoughts, opinions, feelings, and values. Whether we know an elderly person's story or not, we can at least pause for a moment to recognize that there is more *Behind the Old Face*. There is a lifetime of moments and experiences— moments full of joy or devastation, moments of accomplishments and defeats, experiences of love and loss. We experience service and need, laughs and tears, connection and disconnection in our relationships and in the world. We have triumphs and tragedies as well as rewards and consequences of our choices. We must understand that all of these aspects are behind every old face we look into.

As a society, we recognize the beauty and difficulties in aging, and we prepare to care for those who have served us. We prepare for our grandparents, parents, brothers, sisters, aunts, uncles, friends, and ourselves. We prepare for our children and grandchildren, and all the generations to follow, because if we're blessed enough, we will all age.

My vision is to develop communities for aging adults, care providers, and businesses that are self-sufficient and self-contained, based on more of a cooperative model than a traditional business model, but with some aspects of a traditional business included.

The communities include affordable residential living for aging adults, caregiving families, business owners, and health care professionals. They also include health care services, food and goods stores, banks, recreation sites, postal services, environmental services, restaurants, spiritual services, and several common areas scattered throughout the community. The common areas contain buildings of different sizes, including a bigger building with a kitchen and comfortable living areas, and smaller buildings with multiple-purpose areas used for groups and gatherings. There are some comfortable outdoor areas as well, where residents can gather for socialization, picnics, barbeques, and general outdoor enjoyment. Groups are formed based on input and interest from the residents and may include groups for support, interest, education, travel, art, music, fitness, literature, health promotion, family caregivers, and meet-the-neighbors.

The communities are managed by a multi-generational committee of residents comprised of aging adults, care providers, and key business owners and managers who reside in the village. It is preferable for business owners and managers to live in the community, and they will have preferential approval. Those who choose not to reside in the community are required to hire residents as part of their management team, and most if not all employees must be residents.

The communities will be accessible to any aging adults, regardless of income level, as well as care providers, because the housing is affordable for all. Upon considering the community as a place to reside, the individual will meet with the committee to go through an assessment of financial status, skills, and needs. The financial assessment will include current financial status and income needs. The skills assessment will include skills, education, experience, and interests. The needs assessment will include physical, social, and environmental needs.

Assuming the majority of new residents will be recently retired, healthy, active individuals and their caregiving families, the new residents will be placed in the compensation group or volunteer group, based on financial need. The compensation group will fill positions that are fully paid or are performed in exchange for partial or full housing and services. The volunteer group will include individuals who have no need for additional income and will exchange volunteer hours for future service needs.

Caregiving families will also go through the assessment process, including a skills assessment of all children over ten. As an example: a thirty-five-year-old woman who is married with three children ages seven, eleven, and fifteen, and who has been employed as a nurses aide, a licensed practical nurse (LPN), or care provider applies to reside and work in the village. Her husband has a fair-paying job that he likes outside of the village. The woman agrees to work full time as a caregiver in exchange for partial or full housing costs and services. Her husband continues to work outside of the village and volunteers a few hours a week within the village as a residency requirement. Their children are also capable of volunteering a few hours a week. The family may need services such as babysitting or tutoring; they can access those services free of charge in exchange for caregiving work or they can pay for some or all of the services.

A services-and-needs bank will be a necessary part of the cooperative model. As needs change, residents leave, and new residents move in, they will submit the services they can offer and request help with their needs. As services and needs are matched, they are removed from the general services-and-needs fund. As residents age, they will be able to access needed services by paying for them or as an exchange for their work in the community. For example: Alice and John move into the community when John turns sixty-five and Alice is sixty-two. Alice is a retired teacher; John owned a landscaping company. When they move into the village, they do not need additional income. John has Social Security and a retirement fund. Alice collects a decent pension.

After completing their assessments, they are both able to do volunteer work. John is still interested in landscaping, and Alice loves children. John is assigned to work twenty-five hours a week landscaping the common areas and the homes of two elderly residents who are no longer able to do their own yard work. Alice is assigned to provide six hours of tutoring and fourteen hours of child care. They both enjoy working and helping people, so they each offer a couple of additional volunteer hours a week to the main services-and-needs fund.

Alice checks the needs fund and sees that an elderly couple needs some housekeeping help, and an elderly lady needs some minor repairs in her home. She and John volunteer to take those on, and those tasks are removed from the fund.

A few years go by, and John has a stroke. He recovers partially but can no longer provide services to the community. Alice has been working twenty hours a week. She loves what she's doing, but now she needs to be home more because John is unsafe alone and he needs assistance. Alice reduces her volunteer hours to ten hours a week. Someone else is assigned to Alice's childcare duties, and the children she has been tutoring at the common area will come to her home for tutoring. Since John is no longer safe alone, a care provider is assigned to stay with him six hours a week so that Alice can take care of shopping and running errands.

The children in the community can volunteer for a number of jobs, such as emptying trash cans, watering lawns, walking elderly residents' dogs, or conversing with or reading to an aging adult whose spouse needs a bit of respite care. Of course, the assignments will be based on the assessments and will take into consideration age, maturity, interests, and abilities. Training classes can be offered by residents and care providers so that teenagers as well as other residents can learn new skills.

The healthcare within the community will be for minor and common is-sues for which the elderly would normally make a doctor appointment or seek low-priority urgent care. The physicians will include geriatric spe-cialists and family practitioners. Most diagnostic testing, emergencies, surgeries, and other more complex health problems will need to be done in the local hospital.

It will take time to develop and organize the communities as I describe them, but these communities will answer so many needs of aging adults. Further, they will be an incentive for nurses aides and professional caregiv-ers to remain in the profession, and they will attract new care providers.

Many aging adults stay healthy and active. Others are not as fortunate. The inherent needs that bind us are a need to feel valued, a need to have a purpose, and the need to feel a sense of belonging. Many aging adults are socially isolated and suffer from depression. Having a sense of value, belonging, and community would reduce depression. Active, healthy, ag-ing adults want to remain that way, and giving them a sense of purpose and fulfilling work will help them remain healthy for a longer period of time. For so many, when life gets stagnant and unsociable, they begin to decline.

Community provides a type of monitoring. When people are involved with each other in an environment as I describe, and have access to assistance and care, early detection of problems is more likely, which will also con-tribute to reducing healthcare costs. In a cooperative community, nurses and physicians can make house calls, check in on people who are sick, and prevent hospitalizations. Care providers can have easy access to profession-als if they detect illness or some sort of decline; thus, problems can be taken care of much earlier than for people living alone and without assistance.

Cooperative communities will also lessen the need for family caregivers to miss work, reduce work schedules, or leave employment altogether. An estimated fifty million family caregivers are now providing some type of assistance and care to an aging loved one. There is a great cost to businesses from family caregivers attending to aging spouses and parents. MetLife reports those costs to be in the billions of dollars, according to their 2006 report, "The MetLife Caregiving Cost Study: Productivity Losses to U.S. Business." You can find report after report and article after article about the costs and the caregiving crisis. But it's the solutions we need, not more reports and articles.

Raising children in these communities will teach them to value the elderly and the importance of service from a young age, which will most likely continue into their adult lives. The intergenerational approach will benefit all of the residents. There are many studies about the benefits of intergenerational relationships for all parties involved. According to the preeminent developmental psychologist Erik Erikson, developing relationships with the younger generation gives seniors a sense of fulfilment that meets the final stage of social development. Both children and seniors gain a sense of purpose in intergenerational relationships. My husband and I have taken our toddler grandchildren to visit seniors in assisted-living facilities, nursing homes, and hospitals to pass out candy and flowers. The joy on the seniors' faces cannot be described. The joy of giving and seeing all those smiling faces is evident in our grandchildren's faces and their requests to do more visits. If you have small children or grandchildren, you really ought to try spending a couple of hours passing out candy at a local nursing home— keeping in mind sugar-free for diabetics—because it will bring a kind of joy to everyone that can only be understood by experiencing it.

The sense of community among the residents alone will be friendly, caring, and supportive, making it a very pleasant place to reside. These communities will mimic the days gone by when neighbors were neighborly, socialized, and helped each other.

Cooperative communities will encourage people to go into care giving because of the benefits of living in this type of community, where they are able to comfortably live, work, and access services they may not be able to afford otherwise. Like I mentioned, we are facing a crisis like no other with the lack of nurses aides and caregivers. The current low pay, lack of respect, and inability to support themselves deters those who would love the work and do a great job. Those who are in this field leave as soon as they are able to secure a better-paying job. Supplementing experienced and educated caregivers so they could live in comfortable, affordable, and safe housing would attract many into the field.

Seniors will have purpose and feel valued in a community to which they can contribute. Even if they decline as they age, many jobs can be re-aligned to fit in with their restrictions, or new jobs can be assigned. If a resident is no longer capable of performing any work, they already understand that the people who are helping and assisting them will most likely need services in the future as well, so they are less likely to feel like a burden, especially on their families.

This is just a part of the vision I have to meet the needs of aging adults, yet it is a significant part. My main vision is to bring our society to a place of empathy in regards to aging. Unless we all learn and understand what it's like to age, and we seriously take into consideration how we would like to live and be cared for in our older years, we are all facing lives much less desirable than we expect or deserve.

This vision will be the answer to so many issues facing the aging population. No one wants to go to a nursing home. No one wants to live a lonely and invaluable existence. Healthcare costs need to be controlled, care needs are increasing, and most seniors end up moving two to four times following retirement because their needs change. Many retirees downsize their empty-nest home following retirement. When a home becomes too much to care for, assisted living seems like the answer, so another move is made. If they decline to the point of needing more assistance and care, they hire outside care or move to a nursing home. All of this could be avoided in a cooperative living community model.

The cooperative model also helps those unfamiliar with loss of independence to prepare for their own loss or their spouses loss and resulting care needs. Residents won't have to worry and wonder where they'll get care of they need it. Family members won't be under the kind of stress they are now trying to make arrangements for someone to help their parent when they aren't able to provide care or they live too far away. Residents will learn from each other how to better handle the changes that come with aging. Supports will be in place prior to unexpected illnesses and injuries.

As I mentioned, this is a great solution to the shortage of personal care aides. As a previous owner of a homecare agency, I know the struggles of caregivers. Trying to work around children's needs to make a living is difficult enough without mentioning transportation issues, housing issues, and the inability to make ends meet. Caregivers do not make enough money to pay for childcare, so if they lack a reliable family member or friend to attend to their children while they work, they often lose their jobs and too many end up on government assistance. Being a part of a caring community with nice, affordable housing, volunteer child-care providers, and a very limited need for transportation will attract people into the field and allow their children to be raised in a caring, safe environment in which they are taught and expected to contribute, be responsible, and respect the elderly. They will have many successful role models in the elderly residents, which will expand their potential because they will be exposed to all kinds of people, not just the people in the neighborhood they'd typically live in. They will have the opportunity to be tutored so they succeed in school. They will learn about different types of professions and occupations from the elderly residents, which will expand their ability to believe in themselves and what they can do.

Continuous contact within the community will also work as a healthcare monitoring tool, working to get those into the health clinic earlier if a problem is observed rather than later when costs are significantly higher. Nurses aides providing home care are able to monitor nutritional and fluid intake, prevent injuries, assist with medication compliance, assist with activities and exercise, and can report changes early on. This alone plays a major role in reducing healthcare costs, by reducing hospital admissions and readmissions, lowering Medicare's costs for rehabilitation, providing preventive medicine, and catching illnesses and exacerbations of chronic illnesses sooner.

Cooperative communities will save energy by reducing auto usage, limiting auto access within the community, allowing residents to only park in a designated lot at the entrance of the community, and—in warm climates—using only electric golf carts within the community limits. In colder climates, streets and garages behind the structures will keep the community areas free for enjoyment and be safer and more aesthetically pleasing, yet accessible for residents who drive and for emergency vehicles. Sidewalks throughout the community will create a barrier-free opportunity for those who use walkers or canes, or are in wheelchairs. Children can help and play without crossing dangerous roads, and the open environment will encourage community and socialization. Further reductions in energy can be made by using solar and wind power, so it will be less taxing on municipal utilities and save the village and residents money.

Aside from the organization of the cooperative model, the building of the communities wouldn't be much different than current condominium or housing subdivisions. The needs of the majority of the community would require much smaller housing units than are typical of subdivisions today. Most older individuals and couples would be perfectly happy in eight-hundred- or one-thousand-square-foot condominiums or bungalows, which would require much less upkeep and maintenance, keeping those housing costs low.

Although an initial model would take a lot of work and commitment, it would be easily duplicated once the initial village was perfected in its processes. As a fifty-year-old woman who has worked in eldercare and advocacy for over thirty years, I can say that I am not excited to think about living in an assisted living facility or nursing home as I age, and in many ways I dread the thought, but I would welcome moving into a cooperative community. As I think more about this community, I get more excited to move in!

Unless we choose to accept responsibility and focus on creating an alternative model of senior living and care, the current issues, problems, and costs will continue to expand as baby boomers enter their senior years. Isn't it time for an effective and workable solution? Isn't it time we come back to community and sharing life?

I can teach anybody how to get what they want out of life. The problem
is that I can't find anybody who can tell me what they want.
— **Mark Twain**

You've got to think about big things while you're doing small things,
so that all the small things go in the right direction.
— **Alvin Toffler**

Leadership is the capacity to translate vision into reality.
— **Warren Bennis**

We can chart our future clearly and wisely only
when we know the path which has led to the present.
— **Adlai E. Stevenson**

Vision is the art of seeing the invisible.
— **Jonathan Swift**

When you have vision it affects your attitude.
Your attitude is optimistic rather than pessimistic.
— **Charles R. Swindoll**

Dreams are extremely important.
You can't do it unless you can imagine it.
— **George Lucas**

Determine that the thing can and shall be done
and then we shall find the way.
— **Abraham Lincoln**

In the long run men hit only what they aim at.
— **Henry David Thoreau**

Acknowledgements

Nothing Good Happens Alone, and this book and subsequent project is no exception.

I first want to thank and give the glory to God for blessing me with this work and the passion He put in my heart. This book has been written only through Him and the work, passion, gifts, talents, and experiences He has graciously blessed me with.

I thank my husband Bernie who pushed, prodded and loved me with encouragement and support to get this book written and so graciously dealt with all the time I was in my own world thinking and writing. You are such a blessing in my life and I Love You ... Most!

I thank my brother Joe who has always been my biggest cheerleader and supporter! Thanks for believing in me and always making me laugh! You Rock and I Love You!

I want to thank my Mom, Dad, my sister Melanie, brother-in-law Paul, Aunt Cheryl and Uncle Kenny, Uncle Dennis, Gene Rollins, Alan Caldwell, and Wilma Cobb for your very generous financial gifts towards getting this book published. Your gifts and support have made this happen much sooner than possible and touched my heart more than you know. Thank you for your belief in me and the work that is so important. I love you all!

I thank Ron Houghtalin for his friendship, belief, support and the generous gift to begin my work with Jared. Thank you for sharing your family. I love you and your whole family!

Thank you Karl Hauser for the unexpected and extremely generous financial gift towards publishing! You have been a great mentor and person in my life and your generous contribution and support will never be forgotten.

Thank you to Vesper Patrick and NurseTogether.com, Pattie, Casey, Shayne and Tonia at Nurse Talk Radio, Marla and Meg at Winning Life through Pain radio, Alan and Sheila at Everything Elderly radio, Page Cole and all the writers and friends who have publicly supported me and my work.

Jared Rosen, I thank you for believing in this project and intention and showing me a bigger dream than I imagined on my own. I can't thank you enough for everything you have done to make this book a reality! Working with you has been a true honor and I don't know how I would've gotten here without you.

I want to thank Barb Exel for providing interviews at University Living, and always helping me get back to where I need to be with the Lord. You are such a great friend and encourager! I love you lady!

Thank you to Katherine (Kitty) Folker Hamilton and Michelle Mangiapane for your friendship and "teacher's eye" and feedback on the preliminary manuscript.

Thank you to my editor Judith Larson PhD. You did such a great job cleaning up my errors and providing the book's synopsis. You've been wonderful to work with!

Thank you to my cover designer Darlene Swanson. You captured the book in your artwork and the subtleties that covey the message.

My thank you list is not all inclusive of every person who has been a friend, patient, supporter, and encourager along the way or I'd be writing a book of just thank you's!

From my Northridge Church Small Group friends, to my Facebook and Twitter friends, I appreciate every hug, post and bit of support you've given me and my work, so Thank You!

Finally but not last, I thank all my senior friends who opened their lives and heart to me and this book. It has been an honor to know and spend time with you.

To every single supporter who will join in acting on change for a better life for senior's thank you!

I have truly been blessed by all of you and have very deep and heartfelt gratitude for having you all in my life.

With Love and Gratitude,
Angil

Works Cited

University of Michigan; National Poverty Center http://www.npc.umich.edu/
poverty/#2

MetLife; 2011 Market Survey of Long-Term Care Costs http://www.metlife.com/
mmi/research/2011-market-survey-long-term-care-costs.html#findings

The Henry J Kaiser Family Foundation; Total Number of Certified Nursing Facilities,
2010 http://www.statehealthfacts.org/comparemaptable.jsp?cat=8&ind=411

Alzheimer's Association; Facts and Figures 2011 http://www.alz.org/downloads/
Facts_Figures_2011.pdf

California Registry; Residential Care Homes http://www.calregistry.com/housing/
bce.htm

Centers for Disease Control; National Center for Health Statistics http://www.cdc.
gov/nchs/data/hus/hus10.pdf#117

New York Times About.com; Births in the United States 1930 to 2007 http://geogra-
phy.about.com/od/populationgeography/a/babyboom_2.htm

University of Florida IFAS Extension; Developing Intergenerational Relationships
http://edis.ifas.ufl.edu/fy1007

Genworth Care Cost Calculator
http://www.genworth.com/content/non_navigable/corporate/about_gen-
worth/industry_expertise/cost_of_care.html

Resources

There are hundreds of resources on the web, so I'm providing some of my favorites.

AGIS Assist Guide Information Services- http://www.agis.com/default.aspx AGIS has great checklists and information for those caring for a family member, or for professionals to provide resources for families.

AARP Caregiving Resource Center- http://www.aarp.org/home-family/caregiving/ Articles, tools, online support groups and message boards

National Family Caregiver's Association- http://www.nfcacares.org/caregiving_resources/ Tools, resources, statistical information and advocacy.

Caring.com- http://www.caring.com/ Resources, online support groups, experts to answer questions

Family Caregiver Alliance- http://www.caregiver.org/caregiver/jsp/home.jsp great to stay up to date on public policy and advocacy

Medicare- http://www.medicare.gov/default.aspx Check resources on the bottom of the page to find ratings and comparisons on Nursing Homes and Home Health Agencies. I recommend additional diligence in checking out and selecting but this is a good place to narrow down facilities and agencies in your area

Veterans Administration Caregiver Services- http://www.caregiver.va.gov/support_services.asp Services available and VA's Caregiver Support Line – 1-855-260-3274

VA Geriatrics and Extended Care- http://www.va.gov/Geriatrics/Guide/LongTermCare/Eligibility.asp

My Elder Advocate- http://www.myelderadvocate.com/solving-elder-issues/ Help with crisis intervention for nursing home's, evictions, placements, and hospitals.

Alzheimer's Foundation of America- http://www.alzfdn.org/index.htm Education, support, care tips. Grants to offset care costs available http://www.alzfdn.org/AFAServices/aboutAFAgrants.html

The Virtual Dementia Tour® - http://www.genworth.com/content/non_navigable/corporate/about_genworth/industry_expertise/cost_of_care.html The Virtual Dementia Tour® is a scientifically proven method designed to build sensitivity and awareness in individuals caring for those with Dementia. Training is available for individuals and groups.

About the Author

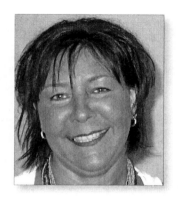

Angil Tarach-Ritchey RN, GCM is an author, speaker, consultant and national expert in senior care. With over 30 years experience in senior care and advocacy Angil is very passionate about eldercare and is well respected in her field.

Angil has written two prior books, **Quick Guide to Understanding Medicare, Medicaid and other payer sources,** available on Amazon Kindle, and **The Aging Question; A Vision for the Coming Elder Boom,** a M2 Ebook which includes video clips of portions of Angil's interviews with Marian and Margaret, available on Dreamsculpt.com. She has written for several websites including NurseTogether, the Alzheimer's Reading Room, Wellsphere, the National Senior Living Provider's Network, Ann Arbor News, and her own blog, Aging in America. Her passion and expertise have led to being published in the Chicago Sun Times, Maturity Matters, Medpedia, Vitamins Health, Medworm, Alzheimer's New Zealand and several other publications. She has been featured on Nurse Talk, WE Magazine for Women; Women on a Mission, Life Goes Strong, You and Me Health Magazine, His Is Mine, and Abec's Small Business Review and quoted in several publications, such as Reuters, Consumer Affairs, PTO Today, Women Entrepreneur and more.

Angil is founder of The Elder Boom™ Foundation. A *501C3 non-profit dedicated to educating families, professional caregivers and healthcare professionals to a new vision of senior living and care. She is available for speaking engagements and consulting at: www.elderboom.org

---

*Pending IRS 501c3 designation at time of publication

CPSIA information can be obtained at www.ICGtesting.com
Printed in the USA
BVOW040226010213

312159BV00003B/11/P